Aids to Undergraduate Medicine

J. L. Burton

MD BSc FRCP

Reader in Dermatology
Bristol Royal Infirmary

FOURTH EDITION

CHURCHILL LIVINGSTONE
EDINBURGH LONDON MELBOURNE AND NEW YORK 1984

CHURCHILL LIVINGSTONE
Medical Division of Longman Group Limited

Distributed in the United States of America by
Churchill Livingstone Inc., 1560 Broadway, New
York, N. Y. 10036, and by associated companies,
branches and representatives throughout the
world.

First Edition 1973
Second Edition 1976
Third Edition 1980
Fourth Edition 1984

ISBN 0 443 03154 1

British Library Cataloguing in Publication Data
Burton, J.L.
    Aids to undergraduate medicine:- 4th ed.
    1. Pathology
    I. Title
    616.07   RB111

Library of Congress Cataloging in Publication Data
Burton, J.L. (John Lloyd)
    Aids to undergraduate medicine.

    Includes index.
    1. Internal medicine — Outlines, syllabi, etc.
I. Title. [DNLM: 1. Medicine — Outlines. W 18 B974a]
RC59.B87   1984   616   83–15276

Printed in Singapore by Selector Printing Co Pte Ltd

Aids to Undergraduate Medicine

Preface

This little book is primarily intended to provide a compact aid to revision for candidates taking the final M B medicine examination, though candidates for other medical examinations may also find it helpful.

Medical educators are unanimous in their condemnation of learning by rote. Nevertheless, candidates in medical examinations still find it necessary to retain a formidable number of facts and I believe that the use of 'skeleton' lists as an adjunct to comprehensive textbooks can encourage an orderly approach to the subject as well as provide a basis for expansion in answers to examination questions.

It is impossible to achieve comprehensive coverage in a book of this size, but I have tried to select information which is worth remembering for use either in the assessment of common clinical situations or in reply to some of the more commonly asked examination questions. Many of the lists I have included are not readily available in the usual undergraduate textbooks, and for some important examination topics I have provided lists which are more detailed than those given in most undergraduate textbooks. Doubtless some readers will be disappointed by the omission of a favourite list and, as a small measure of compensation, there are several blank pages to enable supplementary information to be added according to the personal preferences and needs of the individual.

Most of the lists have been derived from standard specialist texts or medical journals, and where modification has been necessary I accept responsibility for any errors which may have arisen. I should like to thank many of my friends and colleagues, too numerous to mention individually, who have given me much helpful advice and criticism.

In this edition about 25 new lists have been added in response to requests from students, and the section on Management of Medical Emergencies has been considerably enlarged and updated.

1984   J.L.B.

Contents

Hints on the final M.B. medicine examination

> Examinations are formidable even to the best prepared, for
> the greatest fool may ask more than the wisest man can
> answer.
>> Charles C. Colton (1820) *Lacon*, I, 322

The final M.B. examination is intended to prevent the qualification of
incompetent doctors, and the examiners have the duty of ensuring
that every successful candidate is safe to be 'licensed to heal'. They
require to know that:

1. You have a sound knowledge of the basic principles of medicine
   and a common sense approach to the subject
2. You have had practical experience on the wards and can detect
   and interpret physical signs
3. You can prescribe safely, i.e. you know the mode of
   administration and approximate dosage of important drugs, and
   you know their main actions and serious side-effects
4. You can recognize and treat medical emergencies competently

Any candidate who satisfies the examiners on these points is fairly
certain to pass the examination, but bear in mind the lugubrious
corollary that if the examiners demonstrate a deficiency in these
abilities, failure may follow.

REVISION

An important function of revision is to identify and eliminate 'blind
spots'. Nobody can know everything, but you should aim to be
completely ignorant about nothing, and the commoner the topic, the
more you should know about it. A good way to cover topics which
are likely to occur in the examination is to see as many cases on the
wards as possible during your training and to 'read around' them.
Most good physicians base their knowledge on cases they have seen
personally, and it's quite a good idea as a student to keep a brief
record of the patients you have seen as an aid to later revision.

A sound knowledge of medicine is obviously essential, but rapid

1

recall of that knowledge in the exam is equally important. Instead of reading part of the textbooks in detail just before the exam, it's better to refresh your memory of the whole field, even if only in a superficial way. This will be facilitated if your lecture notes are all kept on loose-leaf paper of a standard size so that your knowledge from the various subspecialities can be integrated to avoid confusion and duplication of effort.

ESSAY QUESTIONS

The purpose of an essay question is to discover whether you can assemble your knowledge of a subject, select appropriate facts and opinions, arrange them in an orderly manner and then express yourself with clarity and good style. You should ask yourself what the examiners are trying to test in a particular question. They often have a fairly rigid marking code, awarding marks for each of certain predetermined points that are made, and no extra marks are awarded for even the most fascinating digressions. Candidates rarely fail final M.B. on the essay questions, but those who do are usually failed for not answering the questions that were asked.

Another cause for failure is misjudgement of the time allotted to each question. You should apply the 'law of diminishing returns' as it applies to essay questions — the first 40% for any question is easy, the next 30% is much harder, the next 20% is virtually impossible and the final 10% *is* impossible. Consistency in every question should be your aim. You should not, however, waste too much time on a question which you cannot answer. A blank simply scores no marks but an effusion of rubbish will prejudice the examiner against you.

Where possible questions should be answered in terms of disturbance of physiology. This will demonstrate your knowledge of basic principles and also help you to arrange your answer in an orderly and rational manner.

Many candidates spend hours trying to predict questions by studying old papers. The syllabus is too big for this to be profitable in final M.B., but it's worth checking the type of questions you'll be asked and spending time on any topics on which you are ignorant.

MULTIPLE-CHOICE QUESTIONS

M.C.Q.s are here to stay and you should familiarize yourself with the type of question favoured by your own medical school, particularly since you may be faced with an instruction such as:

'Each question below consists of an assertion (statement) and a reason. On the appropriate line of the answer sheet blacken the space under —

  (a) if both assertion and reason are true and the reason is a correct explanation of the assertion,

(b) if both assertion and reason are true but the reason is not a correct explanation of the assertion,
(c) if the assertion is true but the reason is a false statement,
(d) if the assertion is false but the reason is a true statement,
(e) if both assertion and reason are false statements.'

Many candidates worry about whether they will lose marks for guessing in M.C.Q. exams. It's true that the examiners can adjust scores for the effect of guessing, knowing the number of choices for each question and applying a corrective formula, but the usual correction deducts less than 1 mark for a wrong guess, so unless you are specifically instructed to the contrary it is worth attempting every question. In any case it is a rare question in which you cannot eliminate at least one 'false' answer and whenever you can you have a probability greater than chance of choosing the correct response. Remember too that the words 'always' and 'never' rarely apply to medicine and responses which contain them are unlikely to be true.

Another problem arises when a student has personally seen an unusual case which is the 'exception that proves the rule' and therefore has difficulty in answering an apparently simple question. This is a difficult dilemma, but in general it's probably best to ignore such personally-witnessed rarities unless you have seen them mentioned in standard textbooks.

Shortage of time is rarely a problem in M.C.Q. exams and therefore answers can be checked. In my experience however 'second thoughts' in M.C.Q. exams are rarely an improvement and I think it is preferable to work steadily through the paper once only, but noting any question which will require later thought.

THE CLINICAL EXAMINATION

Examiners rightly lay great stress on 'the clinical' when assessing a candidate and adequate preparation for this part of the examination is vital. The major skill required is of course the ability to elicit physical signs correctly but other factors such as fluency in case presentation and clinical judgement in the interpretation of the signs elicited are also important. The best way to improve your style in 'the clinical' is to obtain regular coaching from a critical senior colleague who will point out your faults. Failing this, you should make arrangements with a fellow student for each to see the other's cases under examination conditions. To obtain the maximum benefit you should of course 'grill' each other on the findings immediately afterwards. This method has the advantage that you will learn to see things from the examiner's point of view and you will quickly come to appreciate those bad habits which commonly cause annoyance to examiners.

Despite current trends, sartorial and tonsorial conservatism is recommended, as both patients and examiners are likely to be middle-aged if not actually senile. Attractive female candidates probably have an advantage but microskirts and low necklines may suggest that the girl who reveals all has something to hide.

THE MAJOR ('LONG') CASE

HISTORY-TAKING

A successful history demands just as much skill as the physical examination, and while two experienced clinicians will usually agree on the physical signs the histories they obtain may be quite different. The examiners realize this and therefore attach more importance to the objective physical findings in assessing a candidate. An accurate history is important for diagnosis, however, particularly with cardiological or neurological patients, who are frequently used as 'long' cases because of their stable physical signs. There is more to the assessment of a cardiological case than merely hearing and interpreting the murmurs, which, contrary to popular belief, are usually 'loud and clear' in examination cases. It is vitally important to obtain the fullest possible details of previous illnesses, especially with regard to the duration, symptoms and treatment of any possible bouts of rheumatic fever, chorea, tonsillitis, SABE, etc., and in female patients you must obtain full details of previous pregnancies. Male patients can often give the results of previous medical grading prior to service in the armed forces, and many patients can give the date and result of previous chest X-rays. Details of the patient's past and present exercise tolerance are of course essential, and you should ascertain from the patient exactly how much physical effort his present work entails. In neurology cases the mode of onset (over minutes, days or weeks), length of history and subsequent course (static, steadily progressive or remitting) will usually suggest the type of pathological lesion present (e.g. vascular, inflammatory, neoplastic or degenerative), and the physical signs will then confirm the anatomical site of the lesion.

When taking a history in exams it is advisable first to list all the patient's symptoms briefly, to discover the type of illness and the systems involved. The symptoms should then be arranged chronologically and full details about each should be obtained. Thus if the patient complains of pain you should determine:

1. The site, with the direction of radiation
2. Its nature and severity
3. Its duration and periodicity
4. Any aggravating or relieving factors
5. Any associated features

Think about the possible diagnosis from the outset and modify your questions accordingly.

Never accept terms such as rheumatism and vertigo at their face value but ask the patient what he means by this. You may be surprised, as was the G.P. who gave several prescriptions for bigger and better laxatives for an old dear who was 'costive', until he discovered she thought this was a synonym for diarrhoea.

Considerable persistence may be needed to prevent the patient digressing. With garrulous patients the previous medical and family histories are particularly difficult to obtain. In such cases stick to essentials and don't hesitate to ask leading questions in order to obtain the necessary information.

The history will allow you to assess the patient's mood, intellect, speech and memory, and you should of course observe the patient closely during the history for signs of dyspnoea, tremor, etc. It is also a good idea on first meeting the patient to ask yourself 'Could this be myxoedema?' as this diagnosis is otherwise easily missed.

EXAMINATION

The ability to elicit and interpret physical signs is of course essential and considerable practice on the wards is required to achieve this skill. A combination of speed and thoroughness is required for exam purposes, and this applies especially to pulmonary percussion, cardiac auscultation and examination of the c.n.s. In auscultation in particular, first impressions are often right and prolonged listening may cause confusion. It's usually more convenient to examine a patient from the head downwards, rather than by systems, and regular practice with an unvarying routine is required if no major points are to be missed. I cannot stress too strongly that people fall their long case not through missing a minor abnormality, but because in their haste they have failed to look for a sign which is in fact present in a gross form. Obvious signs such as a large breast mass, hypertension, marked tracheal shift, gross optic atrophy, unilateral deafness, severe intention tremor, massive splenomegaly, etc. can easily be missed unless the appropriate examination is performed. Such signs may not always be suspected to be present from the history, although it is of course advisable to pay special attention to the systems where you expect positive findings. Thus it would be foolish to accept the absence of a mitral murmur too readily in a patient with dyspnoea, haemoptysis, and a malar flush, or to be satisfied with perfunctory palpation for splenomegaly in a patient with suspected leukaemia.

Equivocal findings can usually be safely ignored unless they are relevant to the symptoms or probable diagnosis. For example it is best not to waste much time over minor degrees of reflex inequality, slight facial asymmetry, impaired vibration sense, etc., unless your patient has a neurological disorder, or a disease which causes a neuropathy. Other common causes of real or imagined equivocation which can often be ignored include slight bilateral pallor or blurring of the optic disc, slight tracheal or apical displacement, soft murmurs and slight inequality of breath sounds. Remember that small differences in percussion are easily imagined and bronchial breathing is uncommon. If a finding is dubious and it doesn't fit, forget it.

For the major case practise working well within the set time limit, so that you have time left at the end to recheck your positive findings and to look again for any associated signs which you might expect to be present in that particular case. Remember that mistakes in the history may occasionally be explained away as being due to the patient's poor memory, but mistakes in the physical signs are entirely the responsibility of the candidate and cannot be condoned.

On completion of the examination you should carefully consider the possible diagnoses and then clarify any doubtful points in the history. You should also amplify the history regarding any unexpected physical signs you have discovered.

Quite apart from any humanitarian considerations it is most important to try to establish a good rapport with your patient. Many of the patients used in the examination are chronic cases with more or less stable physical signs. Since such patients are in frequent demand for teaching purposes they usually have a long experience of young doctors and their difficulties and they are often well aware which of their own physical signs are commonly missed. Occasionally such patients will spontaneously volunteer valuable information with regard to their diagnosis or physical signs, but in other cases a judiciously worded question at the end of your examination such as 'Is there anything else you think I ought to know?' will often prove rewarding. Other useful clues may be obtained by asking the patient to describe the investigations and treatment he has had, and by asking him what he believes to be the cause of his symptoms. Occasionally you'll hit the jackpot with a reply such as 'Well the doctors at Queen Square said it was Frederick Attacks Yer'. You must be prepared for misleading answers however, and these should be ignored if they do not tally with your own assessment of the history and physical signs. These questions should be left until the end as otherwise the replies will prejudice your judgement. Another point to consider is that these questions sometimes provoke in the patient an uncooperative attitude of 'That's for me to know and you to find out' which can make subsequent history-taking difficult.

Before the examiner arrives you should reconsider your diagnosis and ask yourself 'Could this be anything else?' Remember that elderly patients often have multiple pathology, and remember too that although rare diseases occur rarely, their prevalence in examinations is greatly increased. If the diagnosis is uncertain prepare a list of differential diagnoses and consider what investigations you would perform, remembering to mention simple tests such as e.s.r. and chest radiograph before more expensive and possibly dangerous procedures. In most final M.B. exams simple urine tests are required as part of the physical examination of the patient and this important step should not be forgotten. If there is time, you should consider how you would answer probable questions regarding management and prognosis, and in appropriate cases you should try to anticipate what the e.c.g. and radiographs might show.

CASE PRESENTATION

There is quite an art in presenting a case concisely and clearly. The examiners have no time to waste, and hesitant and long-winded presentations are tedious, so you should edit the history, emphasizing important points, leaving out irrelevant detail and giving negatives only if they are important. If the case is straightforward the presentation of the history and examination should form a cohesive account leading to a confident diagnosis. In such cases try to make your assessment as full as you can and say whether the condition in your patient is acute or chronic, mild or severe, simple or with complications. In more difficult cases with conflicting evidence or doubtful signs you will have more reservations, but don't hedge all the time as this irritates examiners and does nothing to conceal your ignorance. Try to make up your mind on the basis of probabilities. Doctors often have to act on the basis of equivocal evidence and the examiners want to see whether you can take a sensible decision.

While it is important to keep your initial presentation concise, it is a mistake to answer the subsequent questions too curtly. The examiner is anxious to see whether you can discuss your patient intelligently and you should try to display your relevant knowledge as much as possible. If anything about the case puzzles you, or there is a problem relating to diagnosis or management, don't be afraid to acknowledge this. If the line of questioning seems to be entering one of your fields of ignorance try to keep the initiative by talking around the subject. With a bit of luck you may introduce a fresh topic that interests the examiner. If he persists in reiterating a particular question this is often because he is trying to establish a very basic point. Examiners can be obtuse in the way they phrase such questions and prolonged silences in such circumstances can be disastrous. Try to talk sensibly around the subject to see what he's aiming at, and with luck a supplementary question will lead you to the required answer.

THE MINOR ('SHORT') CASES

Many students regard the minor cases as a little light relief from the more arduous parts of the examiantion. This is a serious misconception, for the examiners are well aware of the element of luck which enters into the major case, and they attach correspondingly greater importance to the candidate's performance while he is under direct observation. You will be watched as you examine the patient and your style in eliciting physical signs is important. Make a point of positioning the patient properly, and although you should preserve the patient's modesty as far as possible, remember that you may be penalized if you do not get the patient adequately undressed.

As in the long cases, a reasonable compromise must be reached between speed and thoroughness in physical examination, for as a general rule a candidate's score is proportional to the number of cases he has time to examine and diagnose correctly. It is obviously better to err on the side of over-caution rather than to fail because of a major error of omission, but remember that few things irritate an examiner more than the candidate who wastes time performing a tediously meticulous examination in what should be a simple, rapidly diagnosed condition. The examination of the sensory nervous system often provides cause for offence in this respect, and cardiological auscultation presents a similar hazard. If you are unsure of the diagnosis in a case with an 'interesting' murmur, there is usually no point in remaining glued to the patient's praecordium in the hope of being saved by the bell, for the examiner will certainly ask you for a diagnosis before dismissing you. Far better to think quickly, present a sensible differential diagnosis and move on to the next case.

Another important point in the minor cases is to listen carefully to the instructions of the examiner with regard to the part or system to be examined and obey them implicitly. Before recounting your findings however you should always pause and ask yourself whether further examination of more distant parts of the body such as regional lymph nodes, peripheral pulses, finger nails, etc. is required. If you are not clear what the examiner wants you to do, do not be afraid to ask for clarification. For example, if the examiner says 'Examine this patient's heart' it would be reasonable to ask whether he wishes you also to feel the pulse.

The importance of the recognition of clinical associations in the minor cases cannot be overemphasized. In many cases inspection of the patient and his immediate environment as you approach the bed may provide a clue to the diagnosis. For example you may be shown a cutaneous eruption localized to the shin in a patient with exophthalmos (pretibial myxoedema), or you may be asked to give the likely diagnosis of an arthritis in a patient who also has a patch of psoriasis, or marked nail pitting. The key to many minor cases lies in such observations and you should practise looking for such clinical associations until this becomes habitual.

Having elicited the physical signs correctly many candidates fail to be selective enough in applying their knowledge to the particular patient under discussion. Blind application of 'lists of causes' oblivious of the patient's age or sex, the associated physical findings, etc., are guaranteed to create a poor impression. The habit of mentioning rare diseases before common ones is another failing which is easily eradicated with practice.

Hints and tips received from earlier candidates in the short cases are on the whole best ignored. Examiners have been known to change the order of the patients' beds and they will certainly have changed the questions. There is moreover a real danger that you will jump to the diagnosis (which may in any case be wrong) without giving adequate consideration to the differential diagnoses and without eliciting the appropriate physical signs.

It is heartening to realize that for success in the clinical examination omniscience helps, but is by no means essential (indeed a few examiners seem to find it somewhat irritating). More important are adequate practice in examination technique, quick-wittedness, thoroughness, clear enunciation, a confident but modest bearing, and good luck.

THE ORAL EXAMINATION ('VIVA')

The 'viva' tests the depth as well as the breadth of a candidate's knowledge. If he appears to know a topic fairly well the examiners will switch to another subject and if several common topics are satisfactorily dealt with they may go on to test the candidate 'in depth'. For this reason it may be worthwhile for the good candidate to learn about a few unusual multisystem conditions in detail and to try and introduce them into the conversation. For example a student who has spent an elective period in the U.S.A. might choose coccidioidomycosis as a subject to revise in detail. Then if he is asked about pneumonia, meningitis, osteomyelitis, tuberculosis, erythema nodosum or lymphadenopathy he will, after discussing the commoner causes, casually mention coccidioidomycosis. The examiner will often rise to the bait and say 'Ah yes, now what do you know about that?'

The converse of this ploy is that you should not mention anything in the 'viva' unless you're prepared to talk about it. For the same reason you should avoid the use of words such as atelectasis and rales, whose definition is controversial, unless you can discuss the terminology in detail.

You may be given a pathology specimen ('pot') to describe in the viva. Examine it carefully from all sides to try to identify the organ first (not always easy), then describe the pathological lesions you can see, and hazard a diagnosis. If you know the answer try to talk at some length. If you haven't a clue, don't prevaricate but have a guess and go on to the next 'pot'. Tipping it upside down to look at the label is not recommended as it will only make the 'pot' too cloudy to see anything!

If you are shown a radiograph the abnormality is likely to be fairly gross so stand back and take an overall view before looking at the details. Remember that more than one abnormality may be present (e.g. an absent breast shadow with pulmonary metastases, or a

bronchial cancer with rib metastases) so examine the whole film.
Assuming you can spot the abnormality it is best to discuss this from
the outset as examiners get tired of being told that the patient is
slightly rotated and the film is of poor quality.

Finally, have sympathy with your examiner. He cannot be
expected to know everything and if you cross swords with him, give
ground gracefully — after all he may be right!

Cardiology

CYANOSIS

5 g reduced Hb per 100 ml blood produces cyanosis

PERIPHERAL CYANOSIS

Due to poor peripheral circulation

Causes
1. Cardiac failure
2. Vasoconstriction
3. Arterial obstruction

CENTRAL CYANOSIS

Due to inadequate oxygenation

Causes
1. Hypoventilation
2. Lung disease
3. R to L cardiac shunt
4. Decreased PO_2 of inspired gas
   May be simulated by methaemoglobinaemia and sulphaemoglobinaemia

JUGULAR VENOUS PULSE

Height of JVP is measured with reference to sternal angle with
subject at 30° to horizontal
Normally less than 4 cm (vertical height)

CAUSES OF ELEVATED JVP

1. Hyperdynamic circulation:
   (i)   Exercise
   (ii) Fever
   (iii) Anaemia
   (iv) Thyrotoxicosis
   (v)   Pregnancy
   (vi) AV fistulae
2. R ventricular failure
3. Obstruction of superior vena cava (non-pulsatile)
4. Tricuspid stenosis or incompetence
5. Pericardial effusion or constrictive pericarditis
6. Fluid overload (esp. i.v. infusion)
7. Very slow heart rate

P.E.
COPD

TYPES OF ARTERIAL PULSE WAVE

1. **Normal**

2. **Collapsing**
   (i) Aortic incompetence
   (ii) Hyperdynamic circulation ⎰ EXERCISE ⎱ ANAEMIA ⎱ HYPERTH
   (iii) Patent ductus arteriosus
   (iv) Peripheral AV aneurysms
   (v) Arteriosclerotic aorta
   HEART BLOCK -

3. **Plateau**
   Aortic stenosis

4. **Small volume**
   (i) 'Shock'
   (ii) Aortic stenosis   ANY STENOSIS
   (iii) Pericardial effusion
   PULMONARY HT

5. **Bisferiens**
   Combined aortic stenosis and incompetence

6. **Anacrotic**
   Aortic stenosis

7. **Dicrotic**
   Fevers

8. **Pulsus alternans** — Alternate strong and weak beats.
   Left ventricular failure

9. **Pulsus paradoxus** — Volume decreases on inspiration
   (i) Pericardial effusion
   (ii) Constrictive pericarditis
   (iii) Severe asthma
   CB

ARRHYTHMIAS

CLINICAL DIAGNOSIS OF AN ARRHYTHMIA

1. Sinus arrhythmia
Rate increases with inspiration

2. Extrasystoles
Atrial, nodal or ventricular
(i) A premature beat with a compensatory pause followed by a stronger beat
(ii) Usually runs of normal beats occur, but extrasystoles may alternate with normal beats (pulsus bigeminus)
(iii) May disappear during exercise

3. Atrial fibrillation
(i) Completely irregular in time and force
(ii) Worse on exercise
(iii) Carotid compression has no effect
(iv) JVP 'a' waves absent

4. Atrial flutter
(i) Regular radial pulse rate 125–160/min (but can be irregular if there is fluctuating heart block)
(ii) AV block occurs, so that the JVP 'a' waves greatly exceed the pulse rate
(iii) Carotid compression slows the rate while pressure is maintained

5. Paroxysmal tachycardia
Atrial, nodal or ventricular
(i) May be history of previous attacks with sudden onset and cessation
(ii) Carotid compression may decrease the rate even after pressure is relaxed

6. Heart block

Complete (3rd degree)
Heart rate of 36–44/min which does not increase with exercise

2nd degree AV block
May be dropped beats (Wenckebach) or 2:1, 3:1 or 4:1 block. Instability of rhythm is common.

1st degree block
Difficult to identify clinically (PR>0.2 second on e.c.g.)

COMMON CAUSES OF SOME ARRHYTHMIAS

Extrasystoles
1. Idiopathic
2. Fatigue, excessive smoking, alcohol or caffeine ingestion
3. Myocardial ischaemia
4. Digitalis
5. Hyperthyroidism
6. Heart diseases with atrial enlargement (e.g. mitral stenosis)

Paroxysmal tachycardia
1. Myocardial ischaemia
2. Digitalis, especially after potassium depletion

Atrial fibrillation
1. Rh. heart disease, especially mitral stenosis
2. Myocardial ischaemia
3. Hyperthyroidism

4. Drugs eg. O/D Digox
5. Ethanol
6. D. Mellitus

Heart block (all degrees)
1. Myocardial ischaemia
2. Digitalis
3. Chronic heart disease, especially aortic stenosis and congenital lesions
4. Rheumatic fever

APEX BEAT

Heart is enlarged or displaced if apex beat is:

1. Lateral to midclavicular line, or
2. Below 5th intercostal space

   Tapping apex beat indicates RV hypertrophy, but a left parasternal heave is more reliable

Failure to locate the apex beat on palpation
Consider the following possibilities:
1. Excessively fat or muscular chest wall
2. L. pneumothorax, pleural effusion or emphysema
3. Large pericardial effusion
4. Dextrocardia
5. LV hypertrophy. (Remember to feel as far round as the mid-axillary line)

THRILLS

Always indicate an organic defect. The area localizes thee defect

Important causes

Systolic
1. At apex
   (i) Ventricular septal defect
   (ii) Mitral incompetence (rarely)
2. At base on right
   (i) Aortic stenosis
   (ii) Aortic aneurysm
3. At base on left — Congenital heart disease, esp. pulmonary stenosis

Diastolic
At apex — Mitral stenosis

LEFT VENTRICULAR FAILURE

Common causes
1. Myocardial ischaemia
2. Hypertension
3. Aortic stenosis or incompetence
4. Mitral incompetence

Symptoms
1. Exertional dyspnoea
2. Orthopnoea
3. Paroxysmal nocturnal dyspnoea, often with coughing or wheezing
4. Pulmonary oedema (anxiety, dyspnoea, cough and pink frothy sputum)

Signs
1. Tachycardia. May be pulsus alternans
2. Enlarged heart
3. Gallop rhythm
4. May be functional mitral incompetence due to stretched AV ring
5. Crepitations at lung bases. May be rhonchi
6. Cheyne-Stokes respirations may occur in sedated elderly patients

Heart Sounds

I   Very quiet
II   Quiet
III Moderately loud
IV   Loud c̄ thrill
V   Very loud
VI   Deafening

RIGHT VENTRICULAR FAILURE

Common causes
1. Secondary to L ventricular failure
2. Mitral stenosis
3. Cor pulmonale (including pulmonary embolism)
4. Congenital heart disease

Symptoms
1. Tiredness, weakness, anorexia
2. Oedema
3. Gastrointestinal upset. May be hepatic pain

Signs
1. Dependent oedema
2. Elevated JVP
3. May be functional tricuspid incompetence due to stretched AV ring
4. Large tender liver. May be mild jaundice
5. May be ascites or pleural effusion
6. Oliguria by day and nocturia. Urine is concentrated and albuminuria is common
7. Peripheral cyanosis in severe cases

Remember that R and L sided heart failure often appear almost simultaneously

CAUSES OF SYSTEMIC HYPERTENSION

1. Essential
2. Renal disease (especially renal ischaemia)
3. Cushing's disease or glucocorticoid therapy
4. Phaeochromocytoma
5. Primary aldosteronism (Conn's)
6. Coarctation (but B.P. normal in legs)
7. Toxaemia of pregnancy

HEART SOUNDS

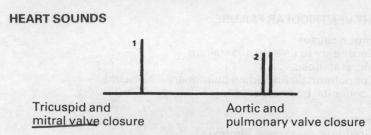

Tricuspid and
mitral valve closure

Aortic and
pulmonary valve closure

N.B.
1. Aortic normally closes before pulmonary
2. Pulmonary closure is delayed by inspiration (due to increased
   venous return caused by decreased intrathoracic pressure)

The normal split therefore widens on inspiration

First sound
Loud in —— APEX
   1. Mitral stenosis
   2. Hyperdynamic circulation
   3. Tachycardia

Soft in
   1. Mitral incompetence
   2. Rheumatic carditis
   3. Severe heart failure

Second sound in aortic area
Loud in systemic hypertension
Soft in aortic stenosis

Second sound in pulmonary area
Loud in pulmonary hypertension
Soft in pulmonary stenosis

Third heart sound

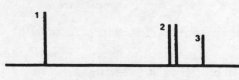

Heard at apex early in
diastole, due to ventricular
distension
Easily confused with
opening snap of mitral
stenosis which is maximal
medial to the apex

Causes
1. Normal in young people (but abnormal after 40)
2. Ventricular failure
3. Constrictive pericarditis
4. Mitral or tricuspid incompetence

(continued)

Fourth heart sound

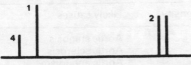

Heard at lower end of sternum late in diastole, due to atrial contraction

Always abnormal, indicates resistance to LV filling

Causes
1. Hypertension
2. Heart block

   Triple rhythm is due to a 3rd or 4th heart sound, or summation of both
   Gallop rhythm is a fast triple rhythm, and indicates actual or incipient heart failure
   Dogmatic pronouncements on the state of the second sound and the presence or absence of the third and fourth sounds are not normally expected of undergraduates

CARDIAC MURMURS

When auscultating, concentrate separately on the heart rhythm, sounds and murmurs. The murmurs most commonly missed in exams are those of aortic incompetence and mitral stenosis. Aortic incompetence is missed either because auscultation was not performed all down the L sternal edge with the patient sitting up at the end of expiration, or because the candidate failed to 'tune in' to the high-pitched murmur. Mitral stenosis is missed either because the patient was not auscultated lying on his left side, or because the candidate listened to only one site in the apical area. A loud first heart sound should suggest the possibility of a mitral stenosis murmur. If several murmurs are present, try to decide which lesion is dominant by consideration of associated clinical features, e.g. in simultaneous AS and AI the pulse may be either 'plateau' or 'collapsing', and in simultaneous MS and MI the presence of a 3rd heart sound with a soft 1st sound suggests the incompetence is dominant.

   If no murmur is heard and the patient gives a history of rheumatic fever, you should exercise the patient and listen again.

   In any patient in whom you suspect rheumatic heart disease you should obtain details of the symptoms, duration and treatment of any previous bouts of possible rheumatic fever, chorea, tonsillitis or bacterial endocarditis.

DIFFERENTIAL DIAGNOSIS OF MURMURS

Timing	Maximal intensity	Likely causes
Ejection systolic	Aortic area	Aortic stenosis Aortic sclerosis Aortic aneurysm Coarctation
	Pulmonary area	Innocent Pulmonary stenosis Atrial septal defect Pulmonary hypertension
	Apex	Innocent Aortic stenosis Aortic sclerosis
Pansystolic	Apex	Mitral incompetence (functional or organic) Ventricular septal defect Fallot's tetrad
	Lower sternal border	Tricuspid incompetence (functional or organic)
Diastolic	Apex	Mitral stenosis
	Lower sternal border	Tricuspid stenosis
	Anywhere along sternal border	Aortic incompetence Pulmonary incompetence Bacterial endocarditis
Continuous ('To and fro')	Cardiac base	Patent ductus arteriosus Simultaneous AS and AI
	Above clavicle	Venous 'hum'

Remember the possibility of extracardiac sounds such as pericarditis

MITRAL STENOSIS

[handwritten: worse the problem the earlier in the murmur in diastole]

Nearly always due to rheumatic heart disease, but rarely may be congenital

Symptoms
1. Progressive exertional dyspnoea
2. Other symptoms of pulmonary congestion:
   (i) Orthopnoea
   (ii) Paroxysmal nocturnal dyspnoea
   (iii) Cough
   (iv) Haemoptysis
3. Acute pulmonary oedema, usually precipitated by exertion or pregnancy
4. Recurrent bronchitis
5. In later stages, symptoms of RV failure (p. 17)

Signs
1. Thin face with purple cheeks ('mitral facies')
2. Pulse may be small volume. May be atrial fibrillation
3. B.P. shows low pulse pressure
4. May be 'tapping' apex beat and L parasternal heave
   May be diastolic thrill
5. 1st heart sound is loud and 'slapping'
   2nd heart sound is loud if pulmonary hypertension is present
   May be 'opening snap' (indicates mobile valve)
6. Rough, rumbling, low-pitched diastolic murmur, localized to the apical area and accentuated by exercise. May be presystolic crescendo if fibrillation absent. Severity of stenosis is indicated by *duration* not loudness of murmur
7. Pulmonary crepitations
8. In later stages, signs of RV failure (p. 17)

Complications
1. Thrombi in L atrium, and systemic embolization
2. Venous thrombosis and pulmonary emboli
3. Subacute bacterial endocarditis (uncommon with atrial fibrillation)

Electrocardiogram
1. May be broad notched P wave
2. May be atrial fibrillation
3. R axis deviation or R ventricular hypertrophy
4. Usually digitalis effects

MITRAL INCOMPETENCE

Symptoms
1. Palpitations and exertional dyspnoea occur early
2. Fatigue and weakness
3. Pulmonary oedema

Signs
1. L ventricular dilatation
2. 1st heart sound is soft and muffled
   3rd heart sound is usual
3. Loud pansystolic murmur, maximal at apex and propagated to
   axilla
   Often obscures 2nd heart sound
4. May be LV failure

AORTIC STENOSIS

Symptoms
1. May be none for years
2. Symptoms of L ventricular failure (p. 16)
3. Syncope or angina on effort

Signs
1. Small volume 'plateau' pulse
2. L ventricular hypertrophy
   May be systolic thrill (best felt with patient sitting forward at end
   of expiration)
3. 2nd sound in aortic area is soft
4. Harsh systolic 'ejection' murmur maximal at aortic area and
   propagated to the neck
5. May be LV failure

Aortic sclerosis murmur is identical, but is distinguished by normal
radial pulse wave and absence of a thrill

Rheumatic Fever

Major : Carditis, Symmetrical nodules, Chorea, Flitting arthropathy
        E. marginatum

Minor : ↑ESR, ↑WCC, ↑ASO, Heart block (1°) β-strep swab
        exquisitely tender joints. Fever

Others Prev. history of strep inf.
        E. nodosum
        Hypochromic normocytic anaemia
        CXR – progressive cardiac enlargement
        Carditis ┬ myocarditis ──── tachycardia
                 │ pericarditis ┬ rub   cardiomegaly
                 │   └ effusion CCF.
                 └ endocarditis ── murmurs eg. carey Coombs

AORTIC INCOMPETENCE

Symptoms
1. May be none for many years
2. Palpitations and dizziness
3. Symptoms of L ventricular failure (p. 16)
4. Angina

Signs
1. Collapsing (Corrigan) pulse. May be visible carotid pulsation or 'head-nodding' or nail bed pulsation
2. B.P. shows wide pulse pressure
3. L ventricular hypertrophy
4. Murmurs:
    (i) Soft high-pitched blowing diastolic murmur down L sternal edge
    (ii) May be a systolic aortic murmur due to increased blood flow
    (iii) May be a diastolic apical murmur (Austin Flint) which simulates mitral stenosis
    (iv) May be 'pistol-shot' noise over femorals synchronous with pulse
    (v) May be diastolic murmur over femorals on slight compression with stethoscope bell
5. May be LV failure

TRICUSPID INCOMPETENCE

Clinical manifestations usually determined by coexisting and predominating mitral stenosis

Symptoms
1. Exertional dyspnoea is common, but orthopnoea and paroxysmal nocturnal dyspnoea are uncommon due to diminished R ventricular output into lungs
2. Gastrointestinal upsets due to venous congestion of GI tract

Signs
1. Elevated JVP with large v waves
2. Pulsatile hepatic enlargement
3. Ascites, which is both chronic and recurrent
4. Peripheral oedema, pleural effusions
5. Pansystolic murmur, maximal near lower sternum, and becoming louder during deep inspiration

CLASSIFICATION OF CONGENITAL HEART DISEASES

CYANOTIC (i.e. R to L shunt)

1. Fallot's tetrad:
   (i) Pulmonary stenosis
   (ii) Ventricular septal defect
   (iii) Over-riding aorta
   (iv) Right ventricular hypertrophy
2. Eisenmenger complex (VSD with pulmonary hypertension)
3. Transposition of great vessels and tricuspid atresia are usually fatal in infancy unless corrected

ACYANOTIC

1. **With L to R shunt**
   (i) Ventricular septal defect
   (ii) Atrial septal defect — usually secundum but rarely septum primum
   (iii) Persistent ductus arteriosus

   These patients may become cyanosed due to cardiac failure, pulmonary infection or severe exercise

2. **With no shunt**
   (i) Coarctation of aorta
   (ii) Pulmonary stenosis — occasionally cyanosed
   (iii) Congenital aortic stenosis
   (iv) Dextrocardia
   (v) Bicuspid aortic valves

Causes of Hypertension = 1° = Essential = 90-95% = Idiopathic

2° - Renal - CGMN, CPN, Polycystic (A.D)

Endocrine - Cushings, Conn's, Phaeochomocytoma Acromegaly, Thyroid ↑

Vascular. Renovascular disease, Renal A. Stenosis Coarctation

Others Pregnancy, Pill

Hypertensive ophthalmology
① AV nipping
② Exudates
③ Haemorrhages
④ Papilloedema.

CAUSES OF SEVERE CHEST PAIN

1. Myocardial ischaemia
   (i) Coronary atheroma, thrombus or vasospasm
   (ii) Aortic valve disease or aortitis
   (iii) Severe anaemia
   (iv) Paroxysmal tachycardia
2. Pericarditis
3. Pleurisy embolism
4. Pulmonary embolism
5. Oesophageal pain (acid reflux, spasm, carcinoma)
6. Chest wall lesions
   (i) Rib fracture
   (ii) Metastatic deposits in ribs
   (iii) Fibrositis or myalgia
   (iv) Herpes zoster
7. Gastric or duodenal ulcer
8. Gallbladder colic
9. Pain referred from thoracic or cervical spine
10. Aortic aneurysm

COMPLICATIONS OF MYOCARDIAL INFARCTION

1. Cardiac arrhythmia
   (i) Sinus or nodal bradycardia
   (ii) Supraventricular tachycardia, atrial flutter, atrial fibrillation
   (iii) Ventricular tachycardia, flutter or fibrillation
   (iv) Heart block . *Intraventricular block.*
   (v) Cardiac asystole
2. Left ventricular failure
3. Hypotension
4. 'Shock'
5. Pulmonary embolism (usually from leg veins)
6. Mural thrombus and systemic emboli
7. Pericarditis
8. Ruptured papillary muscle or chordae tendineae
9. Ventricular septal defect
10. Cardiac aneurysm or rupture
11. Dressler's syndrome (fever, chest pain, pericarditis or pleurisy occurring some weeks after the infarct) *10 days ⇒ 6 weeks*
12. Psychological, including 'L. chest pain'
13. Frozen shoulder and 'shoulder hand' syndrome
14. Iatrogenic; drugs, pacing, etc.

ENZYMES CPK (Pret MB) 2nd day peak
SGOT 3 days post mI
LDH 3-4 days post infarct
Asp transaminase 3-5.

COR PULMONALE

Cardiac disease secondary to chronic disease of lungs or pulmonary vessels

Causes
1. Emphysema and chronic bronchitis
2. Pulmonary fibrosis
3. Multiple pulmonary emboli
4. Severe kyphoscoliosis

Signs of cor pulmonale
1. Warm cyanosed extremities with bounding pulse
2. Raised JVP, hepatomegaly and oedema
3. Triple rhythm and loud P2 due to pulmonary hypertension (but overlying emphysema may cause soft heart sounds)
4. Functional tricuspid incompetence in severe cases

PERICARDITIS

Causes
1. Myocardial infarct
2. Viral (Coxsackie, Echo etc.)
3. Rheumatic fever
4. Pyogenic (pneumonia or septicaemia)
5. Tuberculous
6. Cancer invading the pericardium (bronchus or breast)
7. Severe uraemia
8. SLE, rheumatoid disease

CARDIOMYOPATHY = Any disease of myocardium except infective, ischaemic, backend Hypertensive

CARDIOMYOPATHIES

Congenital   Friedrichs ataxia
              Gargoylism
              Glycogen storage dis
              Pseudohypertrophic MD

Infective — Viral - coxachie
            Bact - diphtheria
                    Endocarditis

Collagen - eg. Systemic sclerosis SLE

Metabolic - Haemochromatosis, Uraemia

Nutritional ← Beri-beri
              Alcohol
              ↓ Protein   Toxic influenza

Endocrine - Thyrotoxicosis
            Acromegaly

Misc.   1° amyloid
        Sarcoid
        Leukaemia
        Endomyocardial fibrosis
        Endocardial fibroelastosis

Idiopathic Subaortic stenosis
Asymmetric Septal Hypertrophy
Hypertrophic Obstructive cardiomyopathy

Electrocardiography

RCA ⇒ inferior infarct + AV nodal damage

LCA ⇒ anteroseptal infarct + Bundle branch
damage.

THE NORMAL ELECTROCARDIOGRAM

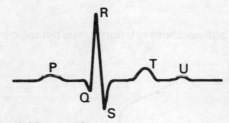

PR should be < 0.20 seconds
QRS should be < 0.12 seconds
1 large square (5 mm) on e.c.g. paper = 0.2 seconds

$$\therefore \text{Ventricular rate/minute} = \frac{300}{\text{No. of large squares between adjacent R peaks}}$$

STANDARD LEADS

E.c.g. interpretation is facilitated by imagining that the standard leads 'look at' the electrical activity of the heart from the following viewpoints in a coronal plane:

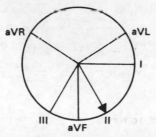

I	Left chest wall
II	Left hip
III	Right hip
aVR	Right shoulder
aVL	Left shoulder
aVF	Perineum

The greatest positive deflection (R wave, due to left ventricular depolarization) is thus normally seen in lead II, and this is the *'cardiac axis'* (see arrow). Right or left axis deviation is thus detected by examining R in the standard leads

MI — 1st - ST elevation
2nd - Q wave appearance
3rd - T wave inversion.

CHEST LEADS

These leads 'look at' the heart in a horizontal plane from the right of the sternum (V1) to the axillary line (V6)

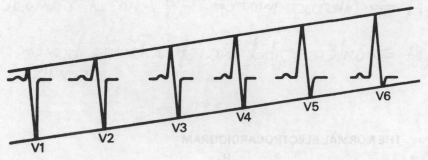

V1   V2   V3   V4   V5   V6

Clockwise or anticlockwise rotation is thus detected by these leads

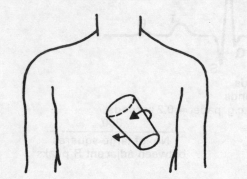

Abnormalities   P wave — Peaked — R.V.H.
                          Bifid — LVH

QRS. — Wide 1. Bundle branch block
                    2. Ventric ectopics

Height — RVH esp V_1 R > S

Q waves — Infarct - Ant - $V_3 + 5$
                           Inf III + aVF

ST segment — Elevation — Acute injury — infarct
                                                  pericarditis

            Depression — Ischaemia

T wave inversion 1. Normal - V_1 (2,3)
                         2. Ischaemia
                         3. L.V.H.
                         4. Bundle branch block
                         5. Digoxin (as c̄ sloping ST depression
                         6. Non - specific

ARRHYTHMIAS

1. Premature beats

Arise from ectopic focus in atrium. AV node or ventricle. Usually followed by 'compensatory pause'.

Supraventricular extrasystole
P is premature and may be bizarrre

Ventricular extrasystole
Bizarre QRS with no preceding P

2. Paroxysmal atrial tachycardia

Normal QRS, but T waves altered by fusion with P waves

PAT with block (usually induced by digitalis). Rapid regular P waves with slower QRS waves

P P   P P

3. Paroxysmal ventricular tachycardia

QRS complexes are slurred and wide but fairly regular. P waves often obscured

4. Atrial fibrillation
Absent P waves and QRS complexes completely irregular

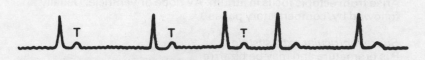

5. Atrial flutter
P waves in 'sawtooth' pattern at 250-350/min and QRS complexes after every 2nd, 3rd or 4th P. The block may fluctuate rapidly, causing QRS to appear irregular

Flutter with 5:1 block

6. Ventricular fibrillation

Rapid bizzare ventricular patterns

HEART BLOCK

Bundle-branch block
QRS exceeds 0.12 seconds with a notched complex

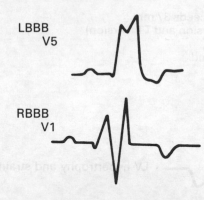

LBBB
V5

M-shaped wave in L chest leads
T wave inversion in lead I

RBBB
V1

M-shaped wave in R chest leads

First degree block
PR interval exceeds 0.20 seconds but rhythm is normal

Second degree block
QRS occurs only after every 2nd, 3rd or 4th P wave
P waves regular, but some obscured by T or QRS complexes

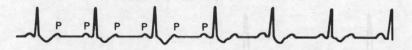

Wenkebach phenomenon
PR interval progressively increases until a QRS is dropped, after
which PR shortens and the cycle is repeated.

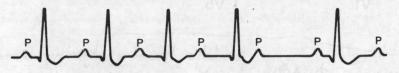

Third degree block (Complete heart block)
P waves and QRS complexes occur completely independently of
each other. Ventricular rate is 25-50/min

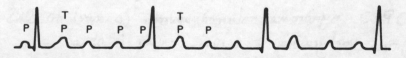

VENTRICULAR HYPERTROPHY

LVH
1. Tall R waves in left chest leads with deep S waves in right chest leads
   Sum of S in VI and R in V5 exceeds 37 mm
2. May be LV 'strain' (ST depression and T inversion)
3. Left axis deviation
4. QRS may be slightly prolonged

± bifid p waves.

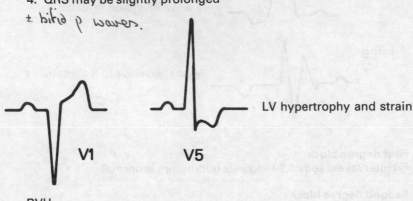

LV hypertrophy and strain

V1   V5

RVH
1. Tall R waves in right chest leads with S waves in left chest leads
2. R axis deviation   ± peaked p waves

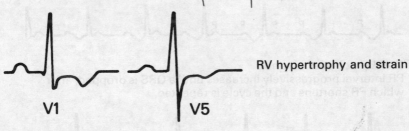

RV hypertrophy and strain

V1   V5

Sinus Bradycardia - athletic training, hypothyroidism, hypothermia, immed post MI, fainting attacks

Sinus tachycardia - Excercises, fear, thyrotoxicosis, pain, haemorrhage.

WPW syndrome - slurred upstroke (Δ wave) to QRS complexes

Atrial tachycardia = ectopic focus in atria

OTHER CAUSES OF E.C.G. CHANGES

MYOCARDIAL INFARCTION

Characteristic changes are:
1. Appearance of Q waves exceeding 0.04 seconds
2. ST elevation and T wave inversion in leads facing the infarct
3. ST depression in leads diametrically opposite the infarct

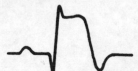

Recent myocardial infarct

Anterior infarct
Usually due to occlusion of the descending L coronary artery. The infarct faces leads I, a VL and the chest leads

Inferior (diaphragmatic) infarct
Faces leads II, III and aVF. Persistence of the acute infarction pattern for more than 6 months suggests ventricular aneurysm

MYOCARDIAL ISCHAEMIA WITHOUT INFARCTION

ST depression and symmetrical T wave inversion

DIGITALIS

Also causes ST depression and T inversion but in a reversed tick pattern

Digitalis also causes:
1. Bradycardia
2. Prolonged PR
3. Shortened QT
4. Any arhythmia, especially bigemini or heart block

HYPOKALAEMIA

ST depression and T wave flattening or inversion. Prominent U waves, which may fuse with the succeeding P

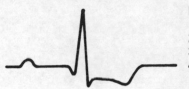

U P

T

ST prolongation

HYPERKALAEMIA

Small P waves with tall peaked T waves
QRS complex widens, and ventricular fibrillation may follow

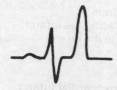

PERICARDITIS

Acute
ST elevation in all the standard leads except aVR, and in most of the chest leads

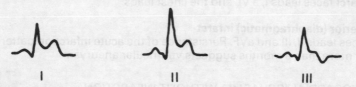

I   II   III

Chronic
ST becomes isoelectric and the T wave flattens and may invert

ACUTE PULMONARY EMBOLISM

1. T wave inversion and Q wave in leads III and V1–V3
2. Transient RBBB
3. Right axis deviation

Tall R in V₁
R = S in V₅ or V₆ rather than V₃

COR PULMONALE

1. Large pointed P waves
2. Changes of RV hypertrophy

Chest disease

LUNG VOLUMES

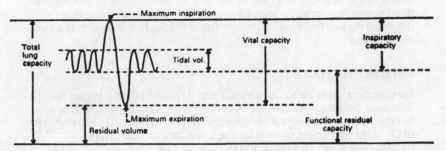

The resting expiratory level is the most constant reference point on the spirometer tracing.

Minute ventilation
Product of tidal volume and number of respirations per minute

Vital capacity
Largest volume a subject can expire after a single maximal inspiration. Normal values increase with size of subject and decrease with age (about 4½ litres in young adult male). Can be reduced in practically any lung or chest wall disease.

Forced vital capacity (FVC)
The vital capacity when the expiration is performed as rapidly as possible

FEV₁
(Forced expiratory volume in one second) — volume expired during first second of FVC

Ratio $\frac{FEV_1}{FVC}$ should be 75% or more, and is reduced in

obstructive airway diseases (asthma, emphysema, bronchitis)

Peak flow
Maximum expiratory flow rate achieved during a forced expiration.
A convenient way to detect a reduction in ventilatory function. Also
useful for serial measurements in the same patient and for assessing
response to bronchial antispasmodics

Residual volume
Obtained by subtracting expiratory reserve volume from functional
residual capacity. Residual volume is normally 20–25% of total lung
capacity but increases in elderly, and in over-inflation of the lungs
(emphysema, asthma)

Anatomical dead space
The volume of air in the mouth, pharynx, trachea and bronchi up to
the terminal bronchioles (about 150 ml). In disease the physiological
dead space may greatly exceed the anatomical dead space due to
the disorders of the ventilation/perfusion ratio, but in health the two
are identical

DIFFUSION DEFECTS

Carbon dioxide is about 20 times more diffusible than oxygen. In
diffusion defects the *arterial Po$_2$* is normal or slightly reduced at rest,
but decreases markedly after exercise due to increased tissue uptake
of O_2. *Arterial Pco$_2$* is normal or even reduced at rest (due to
hyperventilation) and tends to fall on exercise

Causes of reduced diffusing capacity
1. Alveolo-capillary block
    (i) pulmonary oedema
    (ii) pulmonary fibrosis
    (iii) infiltrative lesions, e.g. sarcoidosis
2. Reduction in area available for diffusion
    (i) emphysema
    (ii) multiple pulmonary emboli

Lung compliance
A measure of lung elasticity. Compliance is reduced when the lungs
are abnormally stiff due to pulmonary venous congestion or
infiltrative or fibrotic lesions of the lungs

BLOOD-GAS ANALYSIS

These values must be related to the normal levels expected for the subject, e.g. baby, old man, pregnant woman

Hypoxia
Oxygen deficiency at a specified site

Hypoxaemia
Oxygen deficiency in the blood. In arterial blood of normal resting adult
Pco_2 is about 40 mmHg (4 to 6 kPa)
Po_2 is about 90 to 100 mmHg (12 to 15 kPa)

Causes of hypoxaemia
1. Cardio-respiratory disorders
    (i) Hypoventilation
    (ii) Abnormality of ventilation/perfusion ratio
    (iii) Impaired diffusion
    (iv) Venous to arterial shunt
2. Decreased Po_2 of inspired gas, e.g. high altitude
3. Reduction in active haemoglobin, e.g. coal gas poisoning

Dyspnoea
Subjective awareness of the need for an increased respiratory effort

Hypoventilation
Reduction in lung ventilation sufficient to cause hypercapnia

Kussmaul's breathing (air hunger)
Occurs in acidosis (uraemia, diabetes mellitus) due to stimulation of respiratory centre

Cheyne-Stokes breathing
Amplitude of respiration progressively deepens to a maximum, then decreases to a period of apnoea. Due to diminished sensitivity of respiratory centre to CO_2. Occurs in left ventricular failure, central respiratory depression and in normal infants

OXYGEN THERAPY

In chronic hypoxia due to hypoventilation (e.g. chronic bronchitis, asthma), the arterial Pco_2 is raised and correction of the hypoxia by oxygen in high concentration may release the respiratory centre from its 'anoxic drive' and produce CO_2 narcosis. Low-concentration oxygen masks such as the Ventimask or Edinburgh mask should be used, with serial blood gas analyses.

In hypoxia due to impaired gas exchange (e.g. pneumonia, pulmonary oedema) high concentration masks such as the Polymask are required

Low conc
Edinburg
Ventwi
High conc.
Polymask

HAEMOPTYSIS

COMMON CAUSES

Respiratory
1. Bronchial carcinoma *+ adenoma*
2. Pulmonary tuberculosis
3. Bronchitis
4. Bronchiectasis
5. Lung abscess

Cardiovascular
1. Pulmonary infarct
2. Mitral stenosis
3. Acute left ventricular failure

Less common causes include:
1. Pneumonia, especially pneumococcal
2. Collagen-vascular disease, especially polyarteritis nodosa
3. Idiopathic pulmonary haemosiderosis
4. Bleeding diathesis
5. Mycoses — *ASPERGILLOMA.*
6. Foreign body

Exclude spurious haemoptysis (nasal bleeding, etc.)

In many patients with a small haemoptysis and negative physical findings no cause is ever found despite follow-up with serial chest X-rays

Type of Haemophysis

Frank - Bronchiectasis
Pulm infarct
TB
Mitral Stenosis
Blood stained - Bronial c.a.
Blood streaked - Chronic bronchitis
Bronchial ca.
Rusty sputum - Pneumococcal pneumonia

Complication of pneumonia
Pulmonary - Bronchiectasis
(suppurative pneum
Plewal - Sterile plewal ef
(of staph) → Empyaemia
→ pyopneumothorax
Cardiovascular - Periph. circul.
failure
° bacteraemia
acute pericardi
endocarditis
Neurological - meningism

COMMON CAUSES OF CLUBBING

Respiratory
1. Bronchial carcinoma
2. Chronic pulmonary suppuration

Cystic fibrosis
abscess
empyaema
bronchiectasis.

Cardiovascular
1. Bacterial endocarditis
2. Cyanotic congenital heart disease
3. *Atrial myxoma.*

Less common causes include:
1. Asbestosis, especially with mesothelioma
2. Fibrosing alveolitis
3. Ulcerative colitis
4. Crohn's disease
5. Cirrhosis
6. Thyrotoxicosis (v. rare)   *Thyroid acropachy*
7. Brachial arteriovenous fistula (unilateral)
8. Familial   *Pachydermoperiostosin.*

CAUSES OF PULMONARY COLLAPSE

1. Absorption collapse
Due to complete bronchial obstruction
  (i) Intraluminal, e.g. foreign body, mucus or clot
  (ii) Mural, e.g. bronchial carcinoma or adenoma
  (iii) Extramural, e.g. peribronchial lymphadenopathy or aortic
       aneurysm

2. Pneumothorax or pleural effusion

Remember that in absorption collapse the mediastinum shifts to the
affected side, but in collapse due to air or fluid in the pleural space
the mediastinum may shift to the opposite side

Suppurative pneumonia:-
① Staph pyogenes
② Klebs. pneumoniae
③ Aspiration pneumonia
④ Bact infx of infarcted lung.

Strep pneumoniae
Staph. pyogenes
Strep pyogenes
H. influenzae
Anaerobic streps
Anaerobes
— Vincent spirochaetes.
fusiform bacilli.

δ Dx of pneumonia
P. infarction
TB pleurisy c̄ effusion
Pulm T.B.
Pulmn oedema
Inflam conditions below diaphragm

CAUSES OF PLEURAL EFFUSION

Transudate
(Less than 25 g protein/litre. Implies a systemic cause).
1. Cardiac failure
2. Nephrotic syndrome
3. Hepatic failure

Exudate
(More than 25 g protein/litre. Implies a local cause).
1. Pneumonia
2. Malignancy (bronchial Ca, secondary Ca, Hodgkin's or mesothelioma)
3. TB
4. Pulmonary infarction
5. Collagen-vascular disease (especially SLE)
6. Subphrenic abscess

CAUSES OF PNEUMOTHORAX

1. Traumatic
2. Iatrogenic, e.g. thoracentesis or surgery
3. Spontaneous
   (i) Subpleural bulla
   (ii) Emphysema
   (iii) Asthma
   (iv) TB
   (v) Lung abscess
   (vi) Pneumoconiosis

CAUSES OF EMPYEMA

1. Pneumonia, especially lobar, or secondary to bronchial Ca
2. Lung abscess
3. Subphrenic abscess
4. Mediastinal spesis
5. Chest wound or surgery
6. TB

(handwritten annotations:)

→ Ppt factors Infection, Anaemia, Arrhythmias & Thyroid.

Causes of Congestive H.F. 1. Hypertension 2. Aortic stenosis 3. Coarc
4. Mitral incompetence 5. Aortic incompetence 6. IHD 7. Cardiomyop

Digoxin Rx. 1st day 500 TDS; 2nd 250 TDS, 3rd 250 BD 4th subs 250 D
should ⇒ Old'uns 1st 250 2x; 2nd 125 2x 3rd 62·5 BD 4 " " 62·5
pulse of 70-90 Toxicity Pulse <60 - miss dose. <50 stop drug
NB HYPOKALAEMIA Nausea vomiting diarrhoea
ENHANCES DIGOXIN Colour vision - Red green blurr & halo

CAUSES OF ACUTE PULMONARY OEDEMA

1. *Left heart failure*
   (i) Atrial, e.g. mitral stenosis
   (ii) Ventricular, e.g. hypertension or myocardial infarct
2. *Overload of i.v. fluid*
3. *Inhalation of irritant gas,* e.g. chlorine, dense smoke
4. *Fulminating viral or bacterial pneumonia*
5. *Fat emboli*
6. *Neurogenic* (rare)
   Head injury or cerebro-vascular accident

BRONCHIECTASIS

Dilatation of the bronchi, usually accompanied by recurrent
bronchial suppuration

Pathogenesis
Increased outward traction on the bronchi and weakness of the
bronchial wall due to inflammation are both important

Causes — Congenital eg. Kartageners.
1. Infection
   (i)   Bronchiolitis of infancy
   (ii) Measles or pertussis in children
   (iii) Post broncho-pneumonic collapse in adults
   (iv) Commonly in post-primary TB, but apical, therefore
         secondary infection is unusual
2. Bronchial stenosis or occlusion
   (i)   Adenoma or carcinoma
   (ii) Foreign body or asthma casts
   (iii) Lymphadenopathy
3. Pulmonary aspergillosis
4. Cystic fibrosis
5. Many cases are idiopathic

Clinical features
1. Classical symptom — cough with copious purulent sputum,
   especially on changing posture
2. Classical sign — localized persistent coarse crepitations
3. May be asymptomatic
4. Malaise, intermittent fever, halitosis
5. Weight loss or 'failure to thrive'
6. Dyspnoea, cyanosis or clubbing
7. Haemoptysis ('dry bronchiectasis')
8. Ring shadows on CXR. — honeycomb

COMPLICATIONS OF CA. BRONCHUS

Local effects
1. Bronchial obstruction: collapse, consolidation, abscess
2. Malignant pleural effusion
3. Erosion of large vessel
4. S.V. caval obstruction
5. Direct spread to chest wall, brachial plexus
6. Horner's from cervical sympathetic compression
   Hoarseness from recurrent laryngeal nerve compression
   High diaphragm from phrenic nerve involvement

Metastases
Especially hilar nodes, liver, brain, bone, adrenals

Non-metastatic extra-pulmonary effects
1. Cachexia and anaemia
2. Clubbing (hypertrophic pulmonary osteoarthropathy)
3. Inappropriate ADH → hyponatraemia
   PTH → hypercalcaemia
   ACTH → pigmentation, hypokalaemia, alkalosis
4. Generalised pigmentation or pruritus
5. Neuropathy or myopathy (incl. dermatomyositis)

PNEUMONIA
Anatomical classification
1. *Lobar*
   Due to virulent organisms such as 'epidemic' pneumococcus (e.g.
   Type 3), staphylococcus aureus or Friedlander's (Klebsiella)
2. *Segmental* ('Benign aspiration pneumonia')
   Due to organisms of low virulence
   Often follows upper respiratory tract infections
3. *Lobular* ('Bronchopneumonia' if bilateral)
   Occurs in babies and elderly or debilitated patients. Due to
   haemophilus influenzae, 'carrier' pneumococci, streptococci, TB

Aetiological classification
1. *Infective*
   (i) *Bacterial.* See above. Pneumonia may also be a feature of
       generalized bacterial infections, e.g. brucellosis, typhoid
       fever, plague
   (ii) *Viral*
       a. Ornithosis
       b. Respiratory syncytial
       c. Influenza (usually secondary bacterial infection)
       d. Mumps (usually secondary bacterial infection)
       e. Cytomegalovirus
       f. URT viruses (adenovirus, rhinovirus, parainfluenza)
   (iii) Rickettsial
       a. Typhus
       b. Q fever
   (iv) Mycoplasmal: M. pneumoniae (Eaton agent)
   (v) Yeasts and fungi
       a. Candida
       b. Actinomyces
       c. Histoplasma
   (vi) Protozoa and parasites
       a. Toxoplasma
       b. Amoebae
       c. Pneumocystis carinii

2. *Allergic*
   Collagen-vascular disease (esp polyarteritis nodosa)
   Stevens-Johnson syndrome (erythema multiforme)

3. *Chemical agents*
   (i) Irritant gases: NH_3, SO_2, Cl, oxides of nitrogen
   (ii) Irritant liquids: Vomitus, Lipoid pneumonia

(continued)

4. *Physical agents* — Irradiation

In discussing causes of pneumonia remember the possibility of
1. Pre-existing lung disease, e.g. bronchial carcinoma and bronchiectasis
2. Inhalation pneumonia
    (i) Oral and pharyngeal sepsis and sinusitis
    (ii) Oesophageal obstruction and pharyngeal pouch
    (iii) Alcoholic debauch, drowning or anaesthesia
    (iv) Laryngeal cancer
    (v) Tracheo-oesophageal fistula
3. Predisposing systemic disease such as diabetes, cirrhosis or agranulocytosis.
4. Foreign body not seen on X-ray (e.g. peanut)
5. Acquired immunodeficiency syndrome. Occurs mainly in homosexuals, heroin addicts, Haitians and haemophiliacs.

Complications of pneumococcal lobar pneumonia
1. Pleurisy with effusion, or serous pericarditis
2. Empyema or pericardial suppuration
3. Endocarditis, meningitis (not to be confused with meningismus, in which c.s.f. is normal) or cerebral abscess
4. Delayed resolution
5. Nonspecific complications
    (i) Herpes labialis
    (ii) Septicaemia (may be 'shock')
    (iii) Cardiac failure
    (iv) Cardiac arrhythmia
    (v) Deep vein thrombosis

TUBERCULOSIS

PRIMARY TB

Occurs in subjects never previously exposed to TB
'Primary complex' = Ghon focus + regional lymphadenopathy
Abdominal primary TB and tuberculous cervical lymphadenitis are
now uncommon in the United Kingdom, except in the immigrant
population.

Pulmonary primary TB
Usually heals spontaneously

Complications
1. Local spread in lung
2. Cavitation
3. Pleural effusion (may develop before positive Mantoux)
4. Rupture of caseous node into bronchus causing widespread
   bronchopneumonia
5. Segmental collapse due to bronchial compression by nodes
6. 'Middle lobe syndrome', i.e. bronchiectasis in later life due to
   bronchial compression by nodes
7. Haematogenous metastasis
   (i) Bone
   (ii) Kidney
   (iii) Epididymis or Fallopian tubes
   (iv) Meninges
8. Miliary TB

POST-PRIMARY TB

Reinfection or recrudescence of primary lesion
Usually pulmonary, but may be miliary or atypical in the old or
immunosuppressed.

Pulmonary TB

Complications
1. Caseation ('cold abscess')
2. Bronchogenic spread in lungs
3. Pleurisy
4. Effusion or TB empyema
5. Haemoptysis, may be massive
6. Tension cavity due to valvular obstruction
7. Tuberculoma of lungs
8. Haematogenous metastasis or miliary TB
9. Chronic pulmonary fibrosis and compensatory emphysema (especially in miners)
10. TB tracheitis, laryngitis or stomatitis due to expectoration of mycobacteria
11. Swallowed sputum may cause intestinal TB (usually in lymphoid patches)
12. Amyloidosis

Common presentations of pulmonary TB
1. Asymptomatic (screening CXR)
2. Persistent cough
3. Tiredness, malaise, recurrent coryza, weight loss or fever
4. Pneumonia
5. Haemoptysis
6. Dyspepsia

Note increased incidence in immigrants, elderly, immunosuppressed, diabetic and after gastrectomy for peptic ulcer

CLINICAL FEATURES OF SARCOIDOSIS
1. Bilateral hilar lymphadenopathy (BHL)
   ↓
   BHL + pre-fibrotic pulmonary infiltration
   ↓
   Either resolution or pulmonary fibrosis
2. Constitutional symptoms, erythema nodosum, febrile arthralgia
3. Superficial lymphadenopathy
4. Skin lesions — lupus pernio, infiltrated plaques, nodules, infiltrates in scars
5. Ocular lesions — uveitis, conjunctival infiltrates, etc.
6. Neurological lesions
   (i) Neuropathy, especially facial nerve
   (ii) Meningeal infiltration and local CNS deposits
7. Liver and spleen infiltration
8. Bone involvement, especially phalangeal cysts
9. Hypercalcaemia ± nephrocalcinosis and calculi

DEFINITIONS OF COMMON PULMONARY DISEASE

Simple chronic bronchitis
Chronic or recurrent increase in the volume of mucoid bronchial secretion sufficient to cause expectoration (usually daily cough with sputum for 3 months each year for at least 2 consecutive years)

Chronic obstructive bronchitis
Chronic bronchitis in which there is persistent widespread narrowing of the intra-pulmonary airways, at least on expiration, causing increased resistance to air flow.

Asthma
Is characterized by variable, often paroxysmal, dyspnoea due to widespread narrowing of the bronchioles

Emphysema
Is characterized by enlargement of the air spaces distal to the terminal bronchioles, with destruction of the alveolar walls

Causes of emphysema
A. Localized
   1. Congenital
   2. Compensatory, due to lung collapse, scarring or resection
   3. Partial bronchial occlusion
      (i) foreign body
      (ii) neoplasm
      (iii) peribronchial lymphadenopathy
   4. Rarely unilateral emphysema due to bronchiolitis before age 8 years (Macleod's syndrome)

B. Generalized
   1. Idiopathic (primary)
   2. Secondary to chronic bronchitis,
                      chronic asthma,   } usually centrilobular
      or pneumoconiosis
   3. Senile (physiological)
   4. Rarely familial (some due to $\propto_1$ anti-trypsin deficiency)

SIGNS OF DIFFUSE AIRWAYS OBSTRUCTION WITH LUNG DISTENSION

1. **Inspection**
   (i) Increased A.P. diameter of chest
   (ii) Excavation of supraclavicular fossae during inspiration
   (iii) Jugular venous filling during expiration

2. **Palpation**
   (i) Decreased length of trachea above sternal notch
   (ii) Tracheal descent with inspiration
   (iii) Use of accessory muscles
   (iv) Loss of bucket-handle movement of upper ribs
   (v) Paradoxical movement of costal margin

3. **Percussion**
   (i) Decreased heart and liver dullness

4. **Auscultation**
   (i) Diminished breath sounds
   (ii) Forced expiratory time exceeds 4 seconds

PHYSICAL SIGNS IN LUNG DISEASE

	Chest wall movement	Mediastinum and trachea	Tactile vocal fremitus	Percussion note	Breath sounds	Added sounds
Large pleural effusion	Decreased on affected side	Shift to opposite side	Absent	Stony dull	Absent. May be bronchial (± whispering pectoriloquy) above fluid level	Absent. May be pleural rub above fluid
Consolidation	Decreased on affected side	Central	Increased	Dull	Bronchial	Fine or medium crepitations
Massive collapse	Decreased on affected side	Shift to affected side	Absent	Dull	Decreased	Absent
Fibrosis	Local flattening with decreased movement	Shift to affected side	Increased	Dull	Bronchial	May be coarse crepitations
Large pneumothorax	Decreased on affected side	Shift to opposite side	Decreased	Increased	Decreased	Absent unless bowel sounds are transmitted
Emphysema	Decreased bilaterally ('barrel chest')	Central (except in unilateral emphysema)	Decreased	Increased	Decreased	Absent
Bronchitis	Decreased bilaterally ('barrel chest')	Central	Normal or decreased	Increased	Decreased	Rhonchi and crepitations

Chest X-rays

CAUSES OF WHOLE LUNG OPACITY

1. Consolidation of L lung

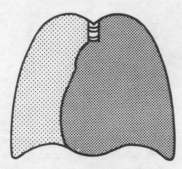

Mediastinum central

2. Massive L pleural effusion

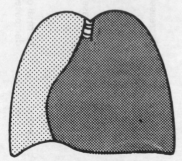

Mediastinum and trachea move to R

3. Collapse of entire L lung

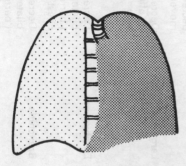

Features
1. Trachea pulled to L
2. R heart border not seen
3. L diaphragm obscured
4. R lung hypertranslucent

Collapse of R upper lobe

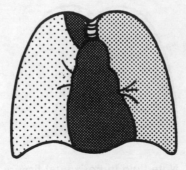

Features
1. Dense wedge against superior mediastinum
2. R hilar vessels drawn up, and widely spaced
3. R lower and middle lobes hypertranslucent
4. Trachea and aortic knob pulled to R

Collapse of L lower lobe

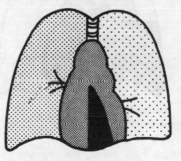

Features
1. Dense wedge in heart shadow
2. L hilar vessels pulled down and widely spaced
3. L upper lobe hypertranslucent

R pleural effusion

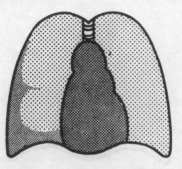

Note fluid in horizontal fissure

R hydropneumothorax

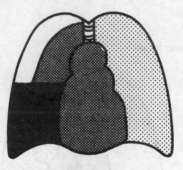

Usually traumatic

Pulmonary oedema

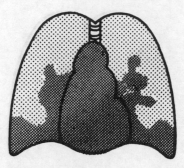

Features
1. 'Bats-wing' shadows-ill defined and confluent, spreading out from hila
2. Generalized lower-zone haze
3. Upper lobe diversion of blood
4. Kerley B lines
5. Enlarged heart

Emphysema

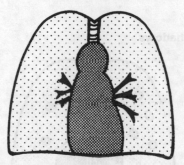

Features
1. Hypertranslucent lung fields
2. Main pulmonary vessels are large, but peripheral vessels are thin
3. Thin vertical heart
4. Horizontal ribs with low flat diaphragm

Single large oval shadow

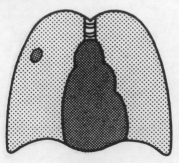

Common causes
1. Bronchial cancer
2. Metastatic deposit, e.g. breast cancer, hypernephroma

Less common causes
3. TB (may be calcified)
4. Abscess
5. Encysted pleural effusion
6. Cyst, e.g. hydatid
7. Adenoma, fibroma or hamartoma
8. AV aneurysm

Multiple circular shadows

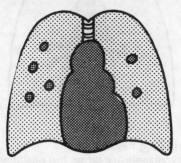

Causes
1. Metastatic malignancy
2. Hydatid cysts
3. Caplan's syndrome (rheumatoid arthritis with pneumoconiosis)

Widespread miliary densities

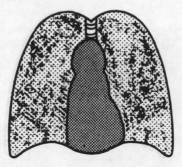

Causes include
1. Miliary TB
2. Pulmonary oedema
3. Bronchopneumonia
4. Pneumoconiosis or haemosiderosis
5. Sarcoidosis
6. Systemic sclerosis
7. Fibrosing alveolitis and rheumatoid lung
8. Hypersensitivity, e.g. allergic alveolitis ('farmer's lung', etc)
9. Neoplasm — Miliary Caymetastases
               Lymphangitis carcinomatosa
               Alveolar cell carcinoma

Bilateral hilar lymphadenopathy

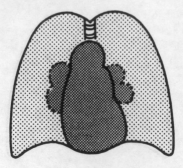

Causes include
1. Sarcoidosis
2. Lymphocytic leukaemia
3. Lymphoma
4. Carcinoma metastases
5. Primary tuberculosis
6. Acute infections, e.g. infectious mononucleosis or whooping-cough

If unilateral, examine lung fields carefully for bronchial carcinoma or Ghon focus

Normal cardiac shadow in PA X-ray

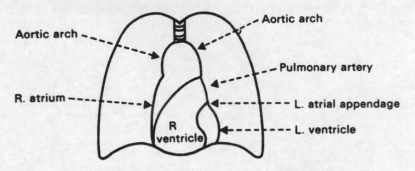

Left atrial enlargement is best seen on R anterior oblique view
Transverse diameter of heart does not normally exceed 50% of chest width

Systemic hypertension

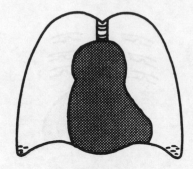

Features
1. Aortic unfolding
2. LV hypertrophy
3. Kerley B lines (horizontal lines in costophrenic angles due to dilated subpleural lymphatics) if LV failure develops

Mitral stenosis

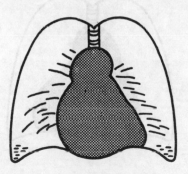

Features
1. Straight L heart border and convex R border
2. Increased pulmonary vascular shadows
3. Kerley B lines

Coarctation of aorta

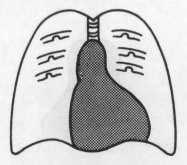

Features
1. LV hypertrophy
2. Small aortic arch
3. Rib notching — esp. Ribs 4→8 (Dock's sign) when classical coarc. — opp. L's arteriosum.

Pericardial effusion

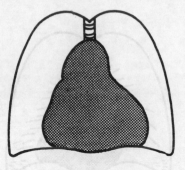

Features
1. Large rounded heart shadow
2. Note sharp cardio-phrenic angles
Distinction from dilated heart may be very difficult

Gallstone presentation

1. Rt upper quadrant pain
2. Incidental finding
3. Obstructive jaundice
4. Flatulent dyspepsia
5. Post-prandial bloating
6. Pancreatitis
7. Finding during investigation into haemolytic anaemia
8. Vitamin K deficiency
9. Gallstone ileus
10. Other fistulae — skin
    - peritoneum
    - colon
    - stomach

Complications of unabating obstructive jaundice

1. > 4/52 — biliary cirrhosis
2. ↑ingly impaired LFT's
3. Suppurative cholangitis

Gastroenterology

CAUSES OF ATROPHIC GLOSSITIS *(SMOOTH RED TONGUE)*

1. Antibiotics
2. Anaemia due to deficiency of Fe, B_{12} or folate
3. Vitamin deficiency (riboflavin or nicotinic acid)

COMMON CAUSES OF SEVERE UPPER GI BLEEDING

1. Duodenal ulcer
2. Oesophageal varices
3. Erosive gastritis
4. Gastric ulcer (may be malignant)
5. Erosive oesophagitis

COMMON CAUSES OF SEVERE LOWER GI BLEEDING

1. Ulcerative colitis
2. Carcinoma of rectum or colon
3. Benign rectal polyps
4. Haemorrhoids or anal fissure
5. Rectal trauma, including biopsy

CAUSES OF DYSPHAGIA

1. **Lesions of mouth or pharynx**
   (i) Stomatitis or glossitis
   (ii) Tonsillitis
   (iii) Quinsy, retropharyngeal abscess
   (iv) Lymphoma of tonsil

2. **Foreign body in pharynx or oesophagus**

3. **Intrinsic disease of pharynx or oesophagus**
   (i) Plummer-Vinson syndrome — iron deficiency, glossitis, pharyngeal web and koilonychia
   (ii) Pharyngeal pouch
   (iii) Inflammation, stricture or neoplasm of oesophagus
   (iv) Systemic sclerosis
   (v) Oesophageal achalasia

4. **Extrinsic compression**
   (i) Tumours in neck
   (ii) Mediastinal tumour, e.g. retrosternal goitre, lymph nodes
   (iii) Bronchial cancer
   (iv) Aortic aneurysm

5. **C.n.s. lesions**
   (i) Bulbar or pseudo-bulbar palsy
   (ii) Myasthenia gravis
   (iii) Congenital muscular incoordination

PEPTIC ULCERS

Differences between gastric and duodenal ulcers

	Gastric	Duodenal
Site	Usually middle 2/3 of lesser curve	Usually duodenal bulb
Gastric acid	Low or normal	Hyperchlorhydria
Pain	After meals	Relieved by meals May occur at about 2 a.m.
Vomiting	Common	Uncommon
Social class	Commoner in lower social classes	Equal prevalence
Pathology	May be benign or malignant	Virtually never malignant

Factors suggesting a gastric ulcer is malignant

Symptoms
1. Anorexia and weight loss
2. Epigastric pain not related to food
3. Dysphagia

Signs
1. Epigastric mass
2. Metastases. Look especially for
   (i) Large irregular liver
   (ii) Supraclavicular nodes (Virchow's) Troisier's sign.
   (iii) Deep vein thrombosis of leg
   (iv) Ascites
   (v) Krukenberg tumour of ovary (felt PR)

Barium metal
1. Filling defect and failure of peristalsis in a site other than middle 2/3 of lesser curve
2. Very large ulcer anywhere in the stomach
3. Leather-bottle stomach

If in doubt gastroscopy and gastric cytology should be performed

Complications of peptic ulcer
1. Bleeding
2. Penetration, e.g. into pancreas, liver or retroperitoneal space
3. Perforation
4. Obstruction
   (i) Oedema and spasm — reversible
   (ii) Cicatricial stenosis — irreversible
5. 'Milk-alkali syndrome' — alkalosis and calcinosis, due to excessive ingestion of milk, alkali and calcium salts

Causes of Chronic hepatic parenchymal disease.
1. Alcohol
2. Infection
3. Metabolic - Wilsons/glycogen storage/ α, anti trypsin b/ Fibrocystic dis
4. Drugs esp αmethyl dopa / methotrexate
5. Cholestasis
6. Congestion.
7. Immunological
8. Malnutrition
9. Cryptogenic cirrhosis

MALABSORPTION
CAUSES

1. **Inadequate digestion**
   (i) Gastric or intestinal resection
   (ii) Hepatic or biliary tract obstruction
   (iii) Pancreatic insufficiency (especially cystic fibrosis)

2. **Parasites or change in intestinal flora**
   (ii) Tape worms
   (ii) Blind-loop syndromes

3. **Intestinal hurry or fistulae**

4. **Coeliac disease**

5. **Tropical sprue**

6. **Intestinal infiltration**
   (i) TB
   (ii) Lymphoma or leukaemia
   (iii) Systemic sclerosis
   (iv) Intestinal lipodystrophy (Whipple's disease)

7. **Enzyme defects**
   (i) Disaccharidase deficiency
   (ii) Hartnup disease

8. **Chronic intestinal ischaemia** e.g. mesenteric atheroma

Clinical features of coeliac disease in adult
1. Loose stools which may or may not be bulky, pale and foul-smelling
2. Weight loss (fat and protein deficiency)
3. Oedema (protein deficiency)
4. Flatulence with distended abdomen (impaired disaccharide hydrolysis)
5. Hypochromic anaemia (Fe deficiency)
6. Macrocytic anaemia (folate or B_{12} deficiency)
7. Peripheral neuritis (B-complex deficiency)
8. Glossitis and stomatitis (B-complex deficiency)
9. Osteomalacia (Ca and vitamin D deficiency)
10. Paraesthesiae, tetany (Ca or Mg deficiency)
11. Haemorrhage (vitamin K deficiency)
12. Muscle flaccidity, arrhythmias (potassium deficiency)
13. Weakness and hypotension (water and electrolyte deficiency)
14. Clubbing

CAUSES OF ASCITES

1. Carcinoma, especially ovarian or alimentary
2. Cirrhosis
3. Hypoalbuminaemia, e.g. nephrotic syndrome
4. Constrictive pericarditis, congestive heart failure
5. Thrombosis or obstruction of inferior vena cava
6. Tuberculous peritonitis
7. Peritonitis in late stages
8. Chylous ascites due to lymphatic obstruction

CAUSES OF OBSTRUCTION OF THE SMALL INTESTINE

The commonest causes are adhesions secondary to operation and bowel incarceration in an internal or external hernia

Mechanical
1. Compression from without:
    (i) Adhesions
    (ii) Fibrous bands
    (iii) Tumours, especially of female pelvic organs
2. Hernia
3. Strictures
    (i) Congenital atresia
    (ii) Acquired:
        Inflammatory
        Neoplastic
        Traumatic
4. Obturation
    (i) Gallstones
    (ii) Faecal impaction
    (iii) Meconium ileus
    (iv) Foreign bodies
    (v) Worms
5. Volvulus
6. Intussusception

Paralytic Ileus
1. Abdominal surgery
2. Peritonitis
3. Acute systemic illness, e.g. pneumonia
4. Painful lumbar conditions, e.g.
    renal colic,
    retroperitoneal haematoma
5. Mesenteric ischaemia
6. Drugs, e.g. ganglion-blockers
7. Hypokalaemia

MEDICAL CAUSES OF ACUTE ABDOMINAL PAIN

1. Food poisoning or dietary indiscretion
2. Peptic ulcer, gastritis, oesophagitis
3. Biliary colic or cholecystitis
4. Pancreatitis
5. Hepatic congestion (hepatitis, cardiac failure)
6. Renal colic, pyelonephritis or cystitis
7. Diverticulitis, ulcerative colitis, Crohn's disease
8. Mesenteric adenitis (children)
9. Mesenteric ischaemia (atheroma, embolism, polyarteritis nodosa)
10. Aortic dissection
11. Gynaecological, e.g.
    Mittelschmerz (ovulation)
    Dysmenorrhoea
    Salpingitis
    Threatened abortion
12. Pain referred from spin or chest (e.g. myocardial infarct)

N.B. Pain in the abdomen which lasts for more than 6 hours without remission is likely to be surgical

DIVERTICULITIS

Clinical features
1. Usually middle-aged or elderly
2. Recurrent bouts of colicky abdominal pain
3. Nausea and vomiting
4. May be either constipation or diarrhoea
5. Tenderness in L iliac fossa, sometimes with a mass

Complications
1. Obstruction due to stricture
2. Perforation
3. Abscess
4. Fistula into bladder or vagina

Ba enema
1. Diverticula may or may not be seen
2. Segmental spasm and irritability of the affected colon (usually sigmoid)
3. Chronic fibrotic deformity

ULCERATIVE COLITIS

Clinical features
1. Commonly presents in 3rd or 4th decade
2. Malaise, weakness, weight loss, pyrexia
3. Chronic diarrhoea, with blood and mucus, which is often severe
4. Pain in L iliac fossa, and rectal tenesmus

Complications
1. Perforation
2. Perianal abscess
3. Acute 'toxic dilatation'
4. Severe haemorrhage
5. Hypokalaemia, hypoproteinaemia, dehydration
6. Skin lesions:
   (i) Pyoderma gangrenosum
   (ii) Aphthous ulcers
   (iii) Erythema nodosum
   (iv) Clubbing
7. Diffuse liver disease
8. Arthritis and uveitis
9. Amyloidosis after chronic abscesses
10. Carcinoma of colon

Ba enema
1. Loss of haustration
2. Straight, narrow, inelastic colon
3. May be 'spicules' due to tiny ulcer craters
4. May be filling defects due to 'pseudopolyps'

Causes of Acute Hepatitis

Infection — Viral — Hep A, Hep B, nonA, non, B. CMV. E.B.V
                       Yellow fever
         Non viral — Leptospirosis icterohemorrhagiae (wiels dis)
                       Toxoplasmosis gondii
                       Coxiella burnetti (Q-fever)
         Incidental — septicaemia

Toxins — ALCOHOL — acute alcoholic hepatitis
                       chronic liver damage
       Phenothiazines / Halothane / Indomethacin / Thiouracil /
       Phenelzine / MAO I / imip - amitriptyline / erythromycin
       isoniazid / rifampicin / chlorpropamide / methyl dopa
         Tetracycline
         Paracetamol
         CCl_4 & Yellow Phosphorus
         Amanita phalloides

Circulatory — Shock & RVF
Others — idiopathic & pregnancy.

CROHN'S DISEASE (REGIONAL ILEITIS)
Clinical features
1. Usually young adults
2. Malaise, weakness, weight loss, pyrexia
3. Intermittent colicky pain in R iliac fossa
4. Mild or moderate diarrhoea
5. Tenderness in R iliac fossa, sometimes with a fixed mass

Complications
1. Obstruction due to stricture
2. Perforation
3. Abscess
4. Fistula into anus, bladder or abdominal wall
5. Fissure-in-ano
6. Malabsorption (especially B_{12})
7. Proctocolitis
8. Erythema nodosum
9. Clubbing

Ba studies (may need both meal and enema)
1. Luminal narrowing of ileum (Kantor's 'string sign')
2. Distorted mucosal pattern
3. 'Skip' lesions

The correlation between radiological appearance and disease activity is often poor

CAUSES OF HEPATOMEGALY
1. Hepatic congestion, e.g. cardiac failure, hepatic vein thrombosis
2. Neoplasm
   (i) Metastases
   (ii) Lymphoma
   (iii) Hepatoma
3. Myeloproliferative disease, e.g. leukaemia, myelofibrosis
4. Infective
   (i) Viral, e.g. hepatitis
   (ii) Bacterial, e.g. Weil's disease
   (iii) Protozoal, e.g. amoebic abscess
   (iv) Parasitic, e.g. hydatid cyst
5. Biliary obstruction
6. Fatty infiltration or early cirrhosis
7. Storage disorders, e.g. amyloidosis, Gaucher's

Causes of Chronic Hepatitis & Cirrhosis
1. Alcohol
2. Infx - Hep B - non-A-non-B
3. Metabolic - Haemochromatosis, Wilson's, α₁ antitrypsin deficit, glycogen storage dis, fibrocystic disease
4. Drugs - methotrexate, methyldopa
5. Cholestasis - 1° biliary - large duct
6. Congestion - Budd Chiari, CCF
7. Immunological
8. Malnutrition
9. Cryptogenic (30%)

CIRRHOSIS

Cirrhosis is characterized by hepatic parenchymal damage with fibrosis and nodular regeneration throughout the liver, accompanied by distortion of the normal lobular pattern

Causes of cirrhosis
1. Cryptogenic (idiopathic)
2. Alcoholism
3. Viral hepatitis (especially serum hepatitis)
4. 'Auto-immune' liver disease — *serum anti-mitochondrial anti-smooth-muscle antibodies high*
   (i) Primary biliary cirrhosis
   (ii) Active chronic hepatitis
5. Haemochromatosis (primary or secondary)
6. Hepato-lenticular degeneration (Wilson's)
7. Hepatotoxins, e.g. methotrexate, carbon tetrachloride

Conditions causing fibrosis but not true cirrhosis
1. Extrahepatic biliary obstruction
2. Chronic venous congestion (e.g. cardiac failure)
3. Schistosomiasis
4. Congenital syphilis

Clinical features of cirrhosis

Features of hepatic failure
1. Firm hepatomegaly in the early stages
2. Low grade fever
3. Skin changes:
   (i) Jaundice in later stages
   (ii) Spiders
   (iii) Palmar erythema
   (iv) White nails
4. Bleeding tendency (decreased coagulation factors)
5. Fatigue, weight loss, dyspepsia
6. Foetor hepaticus
7. Encephalopathy:
   (i) Lethargy
   (ii) Slow, slurred speech
   (iii) Flapping tremor
   (iv) Dementia
   (v) Precoma progressing to delirium and coma
8. Water retention:
   (i) Oedema
   (ii) Hyponatraemia

(continued)

Features of portal hypertension
1. Splenomegaly, often with pancytopenia (hypersplenism)
2. GI bleeding from oesophageal varices
3. Ascites (low plasma albumin is also necessary)

Other features
1. Clubbing
2. Hyperkinetic circulation
3. Sexual changes:
   Females: Erratic menstruation and breast atrophy
   Males: Gynaecomastia, testicular atrophy and scanty body hair
4. Parotid enlargement ⎫
5. Dupuytren's contracture ⎬ in alcoholics
6. Susceptibility to infections ⎭

Causes of cholestasis

1. **Extrahepatic**
   (i) Stone in common bile-duct (CBD)
   (ii) Carcinoma of head of pancreas or biliary tract
   (iii) Pressure on CBD from lymph nodes
   (iv) Stricture of CBD (post-operative or post-inflammatory)
   (v) Developmental anomalies (rare)

2. **Intrahepatic**
   (i) Hepatitis
   (ii) Primary biliary cirrhosis
   (iii) Drugs — Hypersensitivity, e.g. chlorpromazine
                Dose-related, e.g. methyltestosterone
   (iv) Pregnancy or oestrogen ingestion

JAUNDICE

Summary of urinary and faecal bile pigment changes

	Obstructive	Hepatocellular failure with no obstruction	Haemolytic
Urinary bilirubin	Increased	Normal or increased	Normal
Urinary urobilinogen	Decreased	Normal or increased	Increased
Faecal stercobilinogen	Decreased	Normal	Increased

Haematology

ANAEMIA

CAUSES OF ANAEMIA

Deficient RBC production

1. *Deficiency* of:
   (i)   Fe
   (ii) B$_{12}$ or folic acid
   (iii) Vitamin C
   (iv) Protein

2. *Aplastic anaemia*

3. *Marrow infiltration:*
   (i)   Leukaemia
   (ii) Lymphoma, e.g. Hodgkin's
   (iii) Myeloma
   (iv) Myelosclerosis
   (v)   Metastatic carcinoma

4. *'Symptomatic':*
   (i)   Anaemia of chronic infection
   (ii)   Uraemia
   (iii) Liver disease
   (iv)   Hypothyroidism
   (v)   Hypopituitarism
   (vi)   Malignancy
   (vii) Collagen-vascular disease, e.g. SLE, rheumatoid disease

Loss or destruction of RBCs

1. Haemorrhage
2. Haemolysis (p. 71)
3. Hypersplenism

SOME RBC ABNORMALITIES SEEN IN A BLOOD FILM

Size

Anisocytosis
Variation in size, due to anaemia

Macrocytosis
Seen in a film as increased diameter of RBCs, but defined as an
increase in mean corpuscular *volume*

Microcytosis
Defined as a decrease in mean corpuscular *volume*

Shape

Poikilocytosis
Variation in shape, due to anaemia which is usually severe

Spherocytosis
Spheroidal cells seen in hereditary spherocytosis and in acquired *(immune)*
haemolytic anaemia

Elliptocytosis
Elliptical cells. Hereditary. Haemolytic anaemia may or may not
occur

Sickling
Crescentic cells seen when reducing agents act on Hb-S. Hereditary.
Sickle-cell anaemia may or may not occur

Bizarre shapes
Seen in severe uraemia and carcinomatosis

Staining

Hypochromia
Decreased intensity of stain, due to Fe deficiency

Polychromasia
Diffuse basophilia. Indicates active blood regeneration, just as
reticulocytosis does

Punctate basophilia
Stippled appearance seen in severe anaemia or lead poisoning

Target cells (Mexican hat cells)
Occur in:
    (i) Fe deficiency
  (ii) Liver disease
 (iii) After splenectomy
 (iv) Inherited Hb defect, e.g. thalassaemia

CAUSES OF HAEMOLYTIC ANAEMIA

Congenital

1. *Spherocytosis* ('acholuric jaundice')
2. *Haemoglobinopathy:*
   (i) Sickle-cell anaemia
   (ii) Thalassaemia syndromes
3. *Non-spherocytic* (enzyme defects e.g. G6P deficiency)

Acquired

1. *Autoimmune haemolysins:*
   (i) Idiopathic warm or cold antibodies
   (ii) Viral or mycoplasmal infection

2. *Secondary (Symptomatic):*
   (i) Chronic lymphocytic leukaemia
   (ii) Malignant lymphoma
   (iii) SLE
   (iv) Malaria
   (v) Uncommonly—
      Renal disease
      Liver disease
      Carcinoma
      Rheumatoid disease
      TB or syphilis

3. *Drugs and chemicals*, e.g. lead, methyldopa

4. *Haemolytic disease of the newborn*

MACROCYTIC ANAEMIA:

Causes of folic acid deficiency
1. Dietary deficiency or malabsorption
2. Pregnancy
3. Increased cell turnover, e.g. leukaemia or lymphoma
4. Anti-folate drugs, e.g. anticonvulsants

Causes of vitamin B$_{12}$ deficiency
1. Pernicious anaemia or gastrectomy
2. Changed intestinal flora, e.g. blind-loop syndrome
3. Ileal disease, e.g. Crohn's
4. Fish tape-worm (Diphyllobothrium latum)

Other causes of macrocytosis
1. Alcoholism
2. Liver disease
3. Myxoedema

CLINICAL FEATURES OF ADDISONIAN PERNICIOUS ANAEMIA

1. Usually over 30, may have blue eyes, fair hair, premature greying
2. Anaemia of insidious onset
3. Glossitis, often intermittent
4. GI symptoms, e.g. dyspepsia, diarrhoea
5. Subacute combined degeneration
    (i) Peripheral neuropathy
    (ii) Dorso-lateral column involvement
    (iii) Mental changes
    (iv) Rarely optic atrophy, nystagmus, impotence, etc.
        N.B. may be mixed upper motor-neurone and lower motor-neurone signs
6. Mild pyrexia
7. Slight hepatosplenomegaly
8. Retinal haemorrhage
9. Increased incidence of Ca. stomach

LEUCOPENIA

CAUSES OF PANCYTOPENIA

1. Aplastic anaemia (q.v.)
2. Acute leukaemia (in subleukaemic phase)
3. Marrow infiltration:
    (i) Malignant lymphoma
    (ii) Metastatic carcinoma
    (iii) Myelomatosis
    (iv) Myelosclerosis (in late stages)
4. Hypersplenism
5. Pernicious anaemia
6. SLE
7. Rarely, disseminated TB

CAUSES OF NEUTROPENIA SEVERE ENOUGH TO CAUSE SYMPTOMS (AGRANULOCYTOSIS)

1. Aplastic anaemia
    (i) Idiopathic
    (ii) Drugs, e.g.
        cytotoxic drugs
        phenylbutazone
        chloramphenicol
    (iii) Chemicals, e.g. benzene
    (iv) Radiation
2. Selective drug-induced neutropenia (normal Hb and platelets) e.g. thiouracil
3. Acute leukaemia (in subleukaemic phase)
4. Hypersplenism
5. Idiopathic (rare)

LEUCOCYTOSIS

CAUSES OF NEUTROPHIL LEUCOCYTOSIS

1. Bacterial infections
2. Myeloproliferative disease:
   Myeloid leukaemia
   Myelosclerosis
   Polycythaemia vera
3. Haemorrhage, especially internal
4. Tissue damage:
   Trauma (including surgery)
   Burns
   Myocardial infarction
5. Malignancy, especially necrotic tumours and hepatic metastases
6. Drugs, especially steroids
7. Collagen vascular disease e.g. Still's juvenile chronic arthritis

CAUSES OF EOSINOPHILIA

1. **Allergy**
   Hypersensitivity to food or drugs
2. **Parasites**
   e.g. trichiniasis, hydatid
3. **Skin disease**
   (i) Scabies
   (ii) Atopy (eczema, urticaria, hay fever, asthma)
   (iii) Dermatitis herpetiformis

4. **Pulmonary eosinophilia**
   A range of diseases characterized by radiographic pulmonary infiltrates, eosinophilia, and varying degrees of asthma and vasculitis, e.g. Löffler's disease and the pulmonary form of polyarteritis nodosa

5. **Malignancy**
   Especially Hodgkin's disease

POLYCYTHAEMIA

Causes
1. Polycythaemia vera
2. Hypoxia e.g.
   (i) High altitude
   (ii) Cyanotic heart disease
   (iii) Pulmonary disease
   (iv) Obesity
3. Miscellaneous causes of increased erythropoietin, e.g.
   (i) Kidney cyst, neoplasm or hydronephrosis
   (ii) Liver carcinoma
   (iii) Cerebellar haemangioblastoma

Clinical features of polycythaemia vera
1. Headache, dizziness and lassitude
2. Plethoric appearance; engorged conjunctival and retinal vessels
3. Hypertension
4. Splenomegaly
5. Generalized pruritus
6. Dyspepsia due to GI vessel enlargement, or associated peptic ulcer
7. Thrombosis, e.g. cerebral, coronary or mesenteric
8. Haemorrhagic tendency
9. Peripheral ischaemia due to slow circulation or thrombosis
10. Gout

CAUSES OF SPLENOMEGALY

1. Infections especially infectious mononucleosis, septicaemia, bacterial endocarditis and malaria
2. Blood dyscrasis
   (i) Leukaemia (especially chronic myeloid)
   (ii) Haemolytic anaemia
   (iii) Myelosclerosis
   (iv) Polycythaemia vera
3. Malignant lymphoma
4. Portal hypertension
5. Lipoid storage disease
6. Occasionally in rheumatoid disease and SLE

Very large
 CML
 Myelofibrosis
 Malaria
 Kala-azar

Moderate
 Reticuloendothelial dis
  - Hodgekins
  - CLL
 Cirrhosis c̄ portal HT

Slightly - Glandular fever
 Brucella
 Infectios hepatitis
 Subacute septicaemia eg. SBE
Chronic sepsis
Sarcoid
Collagen dis.
Storage dis

ITP
Congenital spherocytosis
Polycythaemia rubra vera

LYMPHADENOPATHY

CAUSES

1. **Infections**
   (i) Focal infection with regional lymphadenopathy, e.g. sepsis, TB, primary chancre
   (ii) Infectious mononucleosis
   (iii) Rubella
   (iv) Secondary syphilis
   (v) Toxoplasmosis
   (vi) Tropical infestation, e.g. filariasis

2. **Lymphoma**
   (i) Hodgkin's
   (ii) Non-Hodgkin's
      a. Follicular
      b. Diffuse

3. **Leukaemia**
   Usually lymphocytic

4. **Malignancy**
   (i) Metastases
   (ii) Reactive changes

5. **Miscellaneous**
   (i) Sarcoidosis
   (ii) Histiocytosis X
   (iii) Chronic inflammatory skin disease
   (iv) Collagen vascular disease, e.g. RA, SLE
   (v) Anticonvulsant drugs

CLINICAL FEATURES OF HODGKIN'S DISEASE

1. Weight loss, malaise, lassitude
2. Fever (the periodic Pel-Ebstein pattern is uncommon)
3. Large, discrete, rubbery superficial lymph nodes
4. Mediastinal or retroperitoneal node involvement
5. Hepatosplenomegaly
6. Pulmonary or pleural infiltration
7. Pain or paralysis due to pressure on nerves or spinal cord
8. Marrow infiltration with pain or pathological fracture
9. Skin:
   Pruritus
   Pigmentation
   Herpes zoster
   Nodular infiltrates
10. Infections due to decreased cell-mediated immunity
11. Alcohol-induced pain

CLINICAL FEATURES OF THE 3 COMMON LEUKAEMIAS

Anaemia, constitutional symptoms (fever, malaise, weight loss) and bleeding (including purpura) occur in all 3 types but are more severe in acute leukaemia and less severe in chronic lymphocytic leukaemia

ACUTE LEUKAEMIA

1. Occurs at any age
2. Onset may be abrupt or insidious
3. Stomatitis and pharyngitis
4. Susceptibility to infections, especially of upper respiratory tract
5. Slight lymphadenopathy
6. Slight or moderate liver and spleen enlargement
7. Bone and joint pain, with sternal tenderness

CHRONIC MYELOID LEUKAEMIA

1. Occurs in middle age
2. Insidious onset
3. Massive splenomegaly
4. Slight lymphadenopathy
5. Moderate hepatomegaly

CHRONIC LYMPHOCYTIC LEUKAEMIA

1. Occurs in late middle age, more often in males
2. Insidious onset, often found accidentally
3. Moderate or marked lymphadenopathy
4. Recurrent chronic infections
5. Moderate liver and spleen enlargement
6. May be haemolytic anaemia
7. Skin lesions:
     (i) Pruritus
    (ii) Herpes zoster
   (iii) Nodular infiltrates
   (iv) l'homme rouge

CLINICAL FEATURES OF MYELOMATOSIS

1. Progressive anaemia
2. Bone pain:
   (i) Osteolytic lesions
   (ii) Pathological fractures
   (iii) Osteomalacia (due to renal phosphate leak)
3. Bleeding, due to thrombocytopenia
4. Fever
5. Renal involvement:
   (i) acute or chronic uraemia
   (ii) Fanconi syndrome
6. Hepatomegaly, occasionally with jaundice
7. Hypercalcaemia
8. Hyperuricaemia
9. Amyloidosis
10. Neuropathy, with raised c.s.f. protein
11. Susceptibility to infections, due to defective antibodies

BLEEDING

May be due to defects of platelets, coagulation or vessels

CAUSES OF THROMBOCYTOPENIA

1. Idiopathic thrombocytopenic purpura (Werlhof's ITP)
2. Causes of pancytopenia (p.   )
3. Drugs causing selective thrombocytopenia, e.g. salicylates
4. Incompatible or massive blood transfusions

   N.B. In thrombocytopenia, bleeding time and capillary fragility are increased, but coagulation time is *normal*

COAGULATION DISORDERS

Congenital

Haemophilias
1. Haemophilia A (VIII deficiency)
2. Haemophilia B (IX deficiency, Christmas disease)
3. von Willebrand's disease (vascular defect + VIII deficiency)

Other congenital deficiences
Factors I, II, V, VII, X, XI, XII or XIII

Acquired
1. Vitamin K deficiency
2. Liver disease
3. Anticoagulant drugs
4. Disseminated intravascular coagulation (consumption coagulopathy)
5. Acute primary fibrinolysis
6. Massive transfusion of stored blood
7. Circulating inhibitors of coagulation

CAUSES OF BLEEDING DUE TO SMALL VESSEL DEFECTS

Congenital
1. Hereditary haemorrhagic telangiectasia (Osler-Weber-Rendu)
2. von Willebrand's disease
3. Pseudo-xanthoma elasticum

Acquired
1. Infection e.g. Bacterial endocarditis, septicaemia, especially meningococcal
2. Drugs e.g. corticosteroids, carbromal
3. Secondary to systemic disease ('symptomatic')
    (i) Cushing's
    (ii) Scurvy
    (iii) Dysproteinaemia
    (iv) Polyarteritis nodosa
4. 'Allergic' vasculitis
    (i) Henoch-Schönlein purpura
    (ii) Cutaneous vasculitis
5. Miscellaneous
    (i) Simple easy bruising
    (ii) Senile purpura
    (iii) Dermatoses, e.g. eczema
    (iv) Fat embolism

Neurology

THE SENSORY SYSTEM

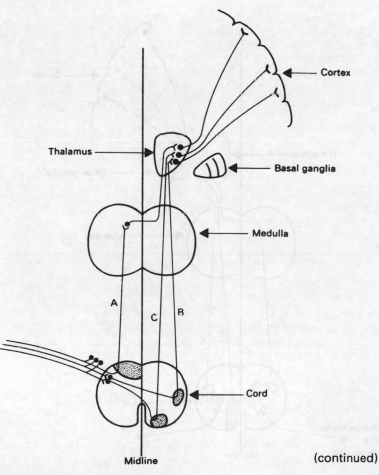

Cortex

Thalamus

Basal ganglia

Medulla

A   C   B

Cord

Midline

(continued)

79

(A) Vibration, proprioception and ½ touch fibres travel via posterior nerve roots up the posterior column without relaying in the cord. They relay in the medulla (nuclei gracilis and cuneatus) and cross the midline to continue as the medial lemniscus to the thalamus. Tertiary fibres travel via the posterior limb of the internal capsule to the sensory cortex (post-central gyrus)

(B) Pain and temperature fibres relay in the cord, cross the midline immediately and travel in the *lateral* spinothalamic tract to the thalamus

(C) Remainder of touch fibres relay and cross the midline in the cord and travel in the *anterior* spinothalamic tract to the thalamus

THE MOTOR SYSTEM

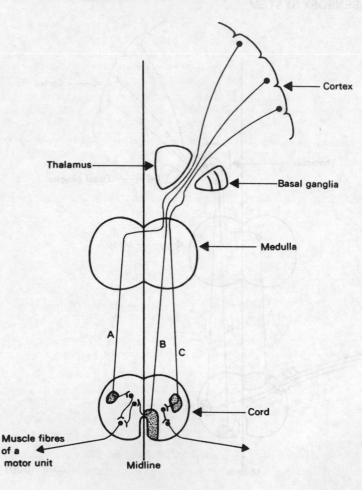

Fibres pass downwards from the motor cortex (pre-central gyrus) into the posterior limb of the internal capsule. In the pons the fibres are scattered, but they regroup in the upper medulla to form protuberances called the pyramids

(A) In the lower medulla the majority of fibres decussate and descend in the *lateral* corticospinal (crossed pyramidal) tracts

(B) Some fibres do not decussate, but descend in the *anterior* corticospinal tract, and then cross in the anterior commissure of the cord

(C) A few fibres descend directly in the *lateral* corticospinal tract with the crossed fibres from the contralateral cortex

Most fibres relay with internuncial cells in the cord, and the anterior horn cells and their fibres then form the 'final common pathway' to the motor end-plates in the muscle. The organization of movement is much more complex than this diagram suggests, since impulses are modified by the cerebellum, the extrapyramidal system and proprioceptive and other sensations

SIGNS OF A LOWER MOTOR NEURONE LESION

1. Weakness and wasting
2. Hypotonicity
3. Decreased reflexes
4. Fasciculation

SIGNS OF AN UPPER MOTOR NEURONE LESION

1. Weakness
2. Spasticity
3. Increased tendon reflexes, with clonus
4. Extensor plantar response

N.B. In pyramidal (UMN) lesions, the extensors are weaker than the flexors in the arms, but the reverse is true in the legs

CRANIAL NERVE SUPPLY

1. **Olfactory**   Smell
2. **Optic**   Vision
3. **Oculomotor**
   (i) All ocular muscles, except superior oblique and lateral rectus
   (ii) Ciliary muscle
   (iii) Sphincter pupillae
   (iv) Levator palpebrae superioris
4. **Trochlear**   Superior oblique muscle
   N.B. Tested by asking patient to look down and *inwards*
5. **Trigeminal**
   (i) Sensory for face, cornea, sinuses, nasal mucosa, teeth, tympanic membrane and anterior two-thirds of tongue
   (ii) Motor to muscles of mastication
6. **Abducens**   Lateral rectus muscle
7. **Facial**
   (i) Motor to scalp and facial muscles of expression
   (ii) Taste in anterior two-thirds of tongue (via chorda tympani)
   (iii) Nerve to stapedius muscle
8. **Auditory**   Auditory and vestibular components
9. **Glossopharyngeal**
   (i) Sensory for posterior one-third of tongue, pharynx and middle ear
   (ii) Taste fibres for posterior one-third of tongue
   (iii) Motor to middle constrictor of pharynx and stylopharyngeus
10. **Vagal**
    (i) Motor to soft palate, larynx and pharynx (from nucleus ambiguus)
    (ii) Sensory and motor for heart, respiratory passages and abdominal viscera (from dorsal nucleus)
11. **Spinal accessory**
    (i) Motor to sternomastoid and trapezius
    (ii) Accessory fibres to vagus
12. **Hypoglossal**   Motor to tongue and hyoid bone depressors

OPTIC PATHWAY

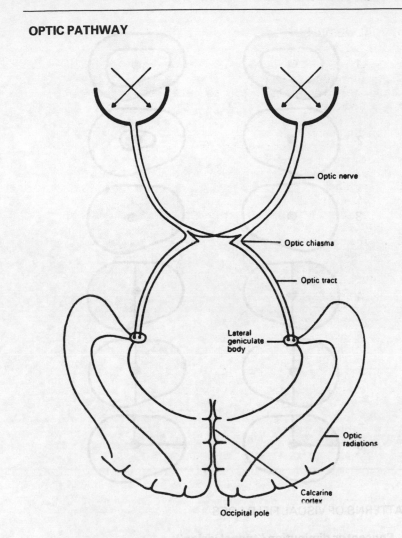

Optic nerve

Optic chiasma

Optic tract

Lateral
geniculate
body

Optic
radiations

Calcarine
cortex

Occipital pole

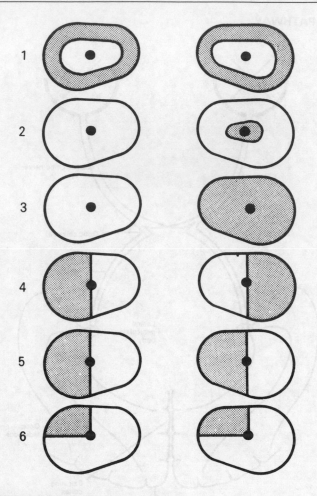

PATTERNS OF VISUAL FIELD LOSS

1. **Concentric diminution ('tunnel vision')**
   e.g. glaucoma

2. **Central scotoma**
   e.g. retinal disease involving macula, retrobulbar neuritis

3. **Complete field loss in one eye**
   e.g. optic nerve lesion

1° adrenal insufficiency

1. Chronic 1° adrenal insufficiency (ADDISON)
   a. Autoimmune adrenalitis ass c pernic anaemie thyroiditis

   b. TB of adrenal gland
   c. 2° tumour
      amyloid
      fungal infx
      haemochromatosis

2. Acute 1° adrenal insufficiency
   a. Any case of 1° adrenal insuffic when stres by infx or Sx
   b. Water-house – Fridrichson syndrome
   c. Iatrogenic – Sx. Anticoagulant o/D.
   d. Breech delivery

2° adrenal insufficiency
   Knackered adenohypophysis.

Acute 1°.
   Vomit / abdo pain / muscular weakness / dehydration confusion coma.

Chronic 1°
   Insidious onset. Tired / Weak / anorexia
Vague abds pains / vomit / wgt loss / dizzy.
      HYPERPIGMENTATION.

S + S of Hyperaldosteronism

Hypertension
   Retinopathy   } rare complications
   Cardiomegaly
Hypokalaemia
Hypernatraemia
Hypochloraemie alkalosis
Glycosuria.

1° Hyperaldosteronism
- Adenoma(ta) } CONN'S SYNDROME
- Idiopathic

2° Hyperaldosteronism (ie ↑ Renin-angio also)
1. Poor renal perfusion
   <u>↓ effective blood volume</u>
   dehydration
   haemorrhage
   loss of sodium & water to extravascular space
   - cardiac failure
     cirrhosis & ascites
     nephrotic syndrome
   salt losing nephritis
   mechanical obstruction of renal artery
   accelerated HT / fibrinoid necrosis
   fibromuscular hyperplasia
   atheroma
   renal arteriolar damage or distortion

2. 1° excess of renin
   Bartter's syndrome (hyperplasia of J-G apparatus

   Renin secreting renal tumours

3. Diuretic therapy.

4. **Bitemporal hemianopia**
   e.g. pituitary tumour

5. **Homonymous hemianopia**
   e.g. tract lesions posterior to chiasma

6. **Quadrantic hemianopia**
   e.g. temporal lobe tumours for superior quadrant
       parietal lobe tumours for inferior quadrant

OPTIC DISORDERS

SQUINTS

Concomitant squint
Due to increased tone in one ocular muscle compared with its synergist. Usually congenital, but may follow an exanthem. Occurs in all neonates

Features
1. Both eyes have full movement if tested separately
2. No diplopia

Paralytic squint
Due to lesions of 3rd, 4th or 6th cranial nerves. Usually causes diplopia

Features
1. 'False' image is always peripheral
2. 'False' image is seen by affected eye
3. Separation of images is maximal in direction of action of affected muscle

3rd cranial nerve (oculomotor) palsy
1. Marked ptosis
2. Eye abducted and depressed
3. Pupil **dilated** and completely non-reactive
   More often partial than complete, especially with lesions near the nucleus

Causes of oculomotor palsy
1. Aneurysm of posterior communicating artery
2. Tumours
3. Brain stem CVA

Cervical sympathetic paralysis (Horner's)
1. Mild ptosis
2. Enophthalmos
3. Pupil **constricted** with no reaction to shading
4. Reduced sweating on ipsilateral half of head and neck
5. Abolition of ciliospinal reflex

   N.B. Everything gets 'smaller'

Causes of Horner's syndrome
1. Carcinoma of apical bronchus (Pancoast's tumour)
2. Cervical sympathectomy
3. Aortic aneurysm
4. Syringobulbia or syringomyelia
5. Brachial plexus lesions (e.g. Klumpke's paralysis)

CAUSES OF PTOSIS
1. Congenital
2. Oculomotor palsy
3. Cervical sympathetic lesion
4. Myasthenia gravis
5. Myopathy

CSF

↑ed IgG in MS, neurosyphilis, neurosarcoid, CTD.

↑ protein — Inf, syph, vasc lesions, tumour, G-B syndrome
diabetes hypothyroidism

↑ cells — bact mening, TB mening, Viral mening, Enceph, syph MS
Glucose ↑ D.M.
→ viral mening
✗ c.a. meningitis, TB
↓ Bact mening

PAPILLOEDEMA

Signs of papilloedema
1. Engorged retinal veins
2. Pink disc with blurred margin
3. Loss of 'cupping'
4. Cribrosa not visible
5. Flame-shaped haemorrhages

Common causes of papilloedema
1. Arterial hypertension
2. Raised intracranial pressure (q.v.)
3. Retinal venous obstruction
   Papillitis (retrobulbar neuritis) is usually due to disseminated sclerosis. It is distinguished by the early severe loss of visual acuity. There may be no fundal abnormality (i.e. 'patient sees nothing, doctor sees nothing')

Causes of raised intracranial pressure
1. Intracranial mass or infection
2. Obstructed c.s.f flow
3. Hypertensive encephalopathy
4. Hypercapnia (CO_2 retention)
5. Pseudo-tumour cerebri
   (i) Thrombosis of intracranial venous sinuses
   (ii) Many rare causes, e.g. oral contraceptives or vitamin A poisoning

CAUSES OF SUDDEN BLINDNESS

1. Retinal detachment
2. Acute glaucoma
3. Vitreous haemorrhage (esp. diabetes)
4. Cranial arteritis
5. Retinal artery or vein thrombosis
6. Migraine (transient)

CAUSES OF FACIAL PARALYSIS

1. **Supranuclear lesions**
   e.g. cerebrovascular accident affecting internal capsule

2. **Nuclear lesions**
   e.g. pontine neoplasm, polio

3. **Infranuclear lesions**
   (i) Cerebello-pontine angle and internal auditory canal, e.g. acoustic neuroma, meningioma
   (ii) Facial canal, e.g. Bell's palsy
   (iii) Extra-cranial, e.g. trauma, parotid neoplasm

In upper motor neurone facial palsy the forehead movements are retained (due to bilateral cortical representation)

DEAFNESS

CAUSES OF DEAFNESS

(A) Conduction deafness
1. Wax or foreign-body
2. Eustachian obstruction
3. Otitis media
4. Otosclerosis
5. Paget's disease

(B) Nerve deafness
1. Traumatic:
   (i) Chronic exposure to loud noise
   (ii) Fracture of petrous temporal bone
2. Infective:
   (i) Congenital syphilis
   (ii) Rubella syndrome
   (iii) Mumps, influenza
3. Toxic:
   (i) Aspirin, quinine
   (ii) Antibiotics, e.g. streptomycin, neomycin
   (iii) Tobacco, alcohol
4. Degenerative:
   Presbyacusis
5. Tumour, e.g. acoustic neuroma
6. Brain-stem lesions (rarely)
7. Rare familial syndromes

RINNE'S TEST:

The ability to hear a tuning fork through air and through the mastoid process are compared. In *normal* people and in *nerve* deafness the air conducted sound is louder, whereas in conduction deafness it is softer

WEBER'S TEST:

The base of the fork is placed on the centre of the forehead; in *nerve* deafness the note is heard in the *normal* ear, whereas in conduction deafness it is heard in the deaf ear

Rinné's +ve = normal. air > bone - Normal
                                    Nerve deafness.

INTRACRANIAL DISORDERS

COMMON INTRACRANIAL NEOPLASMS

Children
Medulloblastoma
Astrocytoma

Adults
Metastatic cancer
Glioma
Meningioma
Acoustic neuroma
Pituitary tumour

Clinical features of intracranial neoplasm
1. Raised intracranial pressure
    (i) Headache, worse on straining and on waking
    (ii) Drowsiness
    (iii) Bradycardia
    (iv) Vomiting
    (v) Papilloedema
2. Progressive loss of neurological function or focal neurological signs (q.v.)
3. Epilepsy
4. Mental symptoms, e.g. personality change, apathy, dementia

Localization of cortical lesions by focal neurological signs

Frontal
1. Mental disturbance
    (i) Dementia
    (ii) Apathy
    (iii) Inappropriate emotion
2. Epilepsy
3. Grasp reflex
4. Unilateral anosmia

Pre-central
1. Jacksonian epilepsy
2. Contralateral spastic hemiplegia

Parietal
1. Sensory disturbance, e.g. lack of 2 point discrimination
2. Visual aphasia
3. Homonymous hemianopia or quadrantanopia (lower)
4. Apraxia
5. Astereognosis

Temporal
1. Anterior lesions — motor aphasia
   Posterior lesions — auditory aphasia
2. Homonymous hemianopia or quadrantanopia (upper)
3. Psychomotor epilepsy

Occipital
Visual field defects

Signs of a cerebellar lesion
1. Intention tremor
2. 'Scanning' speech
3. Nystagmus worse on looking to the side of the lesion
4. Limb ataxia with characteristic gait
5. Hypotonia and pendular reflexes

Vertigo
Ataxia
Nystagmus
Intention tremor
Scanning speech
Hypotonia
Dysdiadochokinesia

Causes of a cerebellar lesion
1. Multiple sclerosis
2. Neoplasms
   (i) In the cerebellum, e.g. medulloblastoma
   (ii) Neuropathy secondary to malignancy such as bronchial carcinoma
3. Cerebellar abscess (often secondary to otitis media)
4. Vertebrobasilar insufficiency
5. Drugs, e.g. alcohol
6. Idiopathic degeneration, e.g. primary cerebellar atrophy
7. Rare hereditary and familial ataxias, e.g. Friedreich's

SUBARACHNOID HAEMORRHAGE

Common causes
1. Ruptured 'berry' aneurysm (85%)
2. Cerebral angioma (10%)

Clinical features
1. Often occurs in middle life
2. Sudden onset of catastrophic headache, usually occipital. Often precipitated by straining
3. Small leakages — delirium or confusion but no loss of consciousness
   Bigger bleeds — vomiting, convulsions and coma
4. Meningism ← S.L. Raising. Kernigs sign Neck stiffness. Photophobia
5. Plantar responses are usually extensor
6. May be slow pulse, or hypertension
7. Occasionally squint, papilloedema, retinal haemorrhage and small sluggish pupils. The characteristic subhyaloid haemorrhage spreads out from the edge of the disc
8. May be pain in back due to blood in spinal theca

CHRONIC SUBDURAL HAEMATOMA

Cause
Rupture of cortical veins as they cross the subdural space. May be traumatic or spontaneous

Clinical features
1. Often elderly patients, after a trivial head injury. Also in infants or alcoholics
2. Latent period of days or months occurs before symptoms develop
3. Gradual onset of headaches, memory loss, dementia, confusion, drowsiness and eventual coma. Symptoms fluctuate from day to day, with lucid intervals
4. May be signs of an intracranial space-occupying lesion, with localizing signs

EXTRADURAL HAEMATOMA

Cause
Fracture of squamous temporal bone with rupture of a branch of the middle meningeal artery

Clinical features
1. Any age, but often young adults with scalp oedema above the ear
2. Concussion may be followed by recovery of consciousness for minutes or hours before the onset of drowsiness and deepening coma
3. Signs of intracranial compression (p.   )
4. Ipsilateral 3rd nerve palsy due to cerebral herniation
5. Progressive contralateral hemiplegia

The signs develop rapidly and immediate operation to relieve the pressure is mandatory

CAUSES OF CEREBRAL INFARCTION

1. Atheroma of intra- or extracranial arteries
2. Cerebral emboli:
   (i) Atrial fibrillation
   (ii) Myocardial infarct
   (iii) Bacterial endocarditis
3. Cerebral ischaemia due to severe hypotension
4. Cerebral arterial spasm, e.g. migraine or following subarachnoid haemorrhage
5. Hypoxia, e.g.
   (i) Cardiac arrest
   (ii) Carbon monoxide poisoning
   (iii) Pulmonary emboli
6. Arteritis, e.g. collagen vascular disease
7. Cerebral thrombosis due to polycythaemia
8. Dissecting aortic aneurysm involving the carotid artery
9. Ligation of carotid artery for intracranial aneurysm

CAUSES OF COMA

1. Syncope (q.v.)
2. Head injury
3. Epilepsy
4. Drugs or toxins (especially alcohol or 'overdose')
5. CVA (Thrombosis, embolism or haemorrhage)
6. Raised intracranial pressure (p. 87)
7. Metabolic
   (i) Hypoglycaemia
   (ii) Diabetic ketoacidaemia
   (iii) Hepatic, renal or adrenal failure
   (iv) Myxoedema
   (v) Electrolyte imbalance
8. Acute c.n.s. infection, e.g. meningitis, encephalitis
9. Acute systemic infection, e.g. septicaemia
10. Hysteria, hypnosis
11. Hypo- or hyperthermia

SYNCOPE ('BLACK-OUT')

A transient loss of consciousness caused by cerebral anoxia, usually due to inadequate blood flow

Causes

1. *Vasovagal*
    (i) Emotion, heat or standing still
    (ii) Loss of blood or plasma
    (iii) Postural hypotension, e.g. drugs or prolonged recumbency
    (iv) Carotid sinus hypersensitivity

2. *Cardiac*
    (i) Stokes-Adams (heart block)
    (ii) Ventricular tachycardia or fibrillation
    (iii) Aortic stenosis
    (iv) Cyanotic congenital heart disease (fall in PO_2)
    (v) Cough syncope (obstructed venous return to heart)

3. *Arterial occlusion*
    (i) Atheroma or embolism (carotid or vertebrobasilar)
    (ii) Cervical spondylosis
    (iii) Strangulation
    (iv) 'Subclavian steal syndrome'

4. *Anoxaemia*
    (i) High altitude
    (ii) Anaemia

CAUSES OF DEMENTIA

PRIMARY PRESENILE OR SENILE DEMENTIA

Idiopathic cerebral atrophy, Alzheimer's, Huntington's etc.

SECONDARY

A. Intra-cranial
1. Tumour, especially frontal
2. Subdural haematoma
3. Vascular, especially atheroma or multiple small emboli
4. Trauma (including concussion in boxers)
5. Infections e.g. encephalitis, neurosyphilis
6. Multiple sclerosis

B. Extra-cranial
1. Metabolic (anoxia, hypoglycaemia, liver failure, renal failure, etc)
2. Hypothyroidism
3. Vitamin deficiency (especially B_{12})
4. Drugs (especially barbiturates)
5. Toxins (especially alcohol, lead)

CAUSES OF PARKINSONISM

1. Idiopathic (especially over 50)
2. Cerebral atheroma
3. Drugs (e.g. phenothiazines)   Wilson's disease
4. Toxins, e.g. manganese, copper, carbon monoxide, kernicterus
5. Post-encephalitic (Encephalitis lethargica outbreaks were in
   1917–1925) » also ∴ coxsackie B » japanese B
6. Head Injury » Punch drunk
7. Tumours compressing midbrain » parasaggital » sphenoidal ridge tumours

CLINICAL FEATURES OF PARKINSONISM

1. Slowness and poverty of spontaneous movement
2. Coarse tremor ('pill-rolling'), with cogwheel rigidity
3. Expressionless, unblinking face
4. Shuffling gait (festination later) with lack of arm-swinging
5. Slurred, monotonous speech and small handwriting
6. Increased salivation and dribbling
7. Oculogyric crises (forced upward deviation of eyes) in
   drug-induced and post-encephalitic types

ABNORMAL GAITS

N.B. Most cases are due to lesions of bone, joint or skin

'Neurological' gaits

1. *Upper motor neurone hemiplegia*
   Arm adducted and internally rotated
   Elbow flexed and pronated
   Fingers flexed
   Foot plantar-flexed, with leg swung in a lateral arc

2. *Spastic paraplegia*
   Stiff jerky 'scissors' gait, with complicated assisting movements
   of upper limbs

3. *Parkinsonism*
   Small shuffling hurried steps
   Flexion of neck, elbows, wrists and MP joints with thumbs
   adducted

4. *Cerebellar lesion*
   'Drunken' gait on a broad base. Feet raised excessively and
   placed carefully, with patient looking ahead. Tends to fall to side
   of lesion

5. *Posterior column lesion*
   Patient walks on a broad base but bangs feet down clumsily and
   tends to look at feet. Rombergism is present

6. *High-stepping gait*
   Due to foot drop

7. *Proximal myopathy*
   Waddling gait with broad base, lordosis and marked body swing.
   This gait occurs also in congenital hip dislocation and pregnancy

8. *Hysterical*
   Usually bizarre and inconsistent, and the patient rarely falls

9. *Involuntary movements*
   (i) *Choreiform* — Jerky movements of short duration, affecting
       limbs and face
   (ii) *Athetoid* — Slow writhing of arms and legs with flexed
        fingers, thumb and wrist
   (iii) *Dystonia musculorum* (torsion spasm) — Intense sustained
         spasm of proximal and trunk muscles may cause bizarre
         stepping or bowing of the trunk
   (iv) *Hemiballismus* — Unilateral forceful throwing movements
        which are almost continuous

CLASSIFICATION OF SPEECH DEFECTS

1. Dysphasia (disorder in use of symbols for communication whether spoken, heard, written or read)
2. Dysarthria (disorder of articulation) *slurring of syllables & consonant*
3. Dysphonia (disorder of vocalization)
4. Dementia (intellectual deterioration)

Causes of dysphasia
1. Motor — due to lesion of inferior frontal gyrus of dominant frontal lobe. (Broca's area)
2. Sensory — due to lesion of dominant temporoparietal cortex

Causes of dysarthria
1. Bulbar or pseudo-bulbar palsy
2. Basal ganglia lesions
3. Cerebellar lesions *-(scanning dysarthria)*
4. Weakness or paralysis of facial muscles
5. Oral lesions including loose dentures

Causes of dysphonia
1. Functional (hysteria)
2. Lesions of recurrent laryngeal nerve (Ca. bronchus, aortic aneurysm)
3. Vocal cord lesion (infection, tumour, etc.)

SPINAL CORD COMPRESSION

Symptoms
1. Root pains occur early. Often precipitated by movement or straining
2. Progressive weakness, paraesthesiae and sensory loss
3. Sphincter disturbances occur at a late stage

Signs
1. Lower motor neurone signs at level of compression and spasticity below
2. Sensory or reflex 'level'. May be hyperaesthesia at the affected level
3. Loss of abdominal reflexes in thoracic or cervical lesions

Causes of cord compression

1. *Vertebral*
   (i) Metastatic cancer (esp. bronchus, breast, prostate)
   (ii) Osteoporotic collapse
   (iii) Pott's disease (TB)
   (iv) Spondylosis with disc prolapse

2. *Extra-dural*
   (i) Abscess

3. *Intra-dural*
   (i) Infiltration of meninges — lymphoma, leukaemia
   (ii) Extra-medullary tumours — meningioma, neurofibroma
   (iii) Intra-medullary tumours — glioma

Causes of root lesions
1. Disc protrusion
2. Spondylosis (osteophyte)
3. Metastatic cancer

Clinical features of root lesions
1. Pain in the appropriate myotome, aggravated by straining
2. Paraesthesiae in the dermatome
3. Spinal muscle spasm, e.g. lumbar scoliosis or restriction of neck movement
4. Weakness, wasting and fasciculation of the myotome, with decreased tendon reflex

Myotomes worth remembering
C6 — Biceps, brachioradialis, radial extensors of wrist
C7 — Triceps, ulnar extensors of wrist, finger extensors
C8 — Finger flexors
L4 — Quadriceps femoris
L5 — Extensor hallucis longus
S1 — Plantar flexors

SYRINGOMYELIA AND SYRINGOBULBIA

Syringomyelia

Usually starts in base of posterior horn of cervical region

Clinical features
Insidious onset of
1. Weakness and wasting of small muscles of hand
2. Dissociated sensory loss in hand (pain and temperature only)
3. Trophic changes:
   (i) Cyanosis of fingers
   (ii) Ulceration and scarring
   (iii) Swollen fingers due to subcutaneous hypertrophy
4. Loss of tendon reflexes
5. Painful arm
6. Spastic paraplegia
7. Charcot joints (neck and shoulders)

Syringobulbia

Medulla may be initial site, or may be involved by upward extension
from cord

Clinical features
1. Facial pain or sensory loss (Cr. 5)
2. Vertigo and nystagmus (Cr. 8)
3. Facial, palatal or laryngeal palsy (Cr. 7, 9, 10, 11)
4. Wasted tongue (Cr. 12)
5. Horner's syndrome (Sympathetic)

BULBAR PALSY

Bilateral *lower* motor neurone lesions of the bulbar nuclei (9, 10, 11
and 12 with lowermost part of 7)

Clinical features
1. Dysarthria
2. Dysphagia, especially with fluids
3. Wasted fibrillating tongue
4. Palatal paralysis

Causes
1. Motor neurone disease
2. Polio
3. Encephalitis
4. Syringobulbia

PSEUDO-BULBAR PALSY

Bilateral *upper* motor neurone lesions of the same nuclei

Clinical features
1. Dysarthria
2. Dysphagia
3. Spastic tongue
4. Exaggerated jaw-jerk (spastic masseters)
5. Emotional lability

Causes
1. Ischaemia of internal capsule
2. Motor neurone disease
3. Disseminated sclerosis

PERIPHERAL NEUROPATHY

Characterized by symmetrical flaccid weakness and sensory changes of 'glove and stocking' distribution

Causes of polyneuropathy

1. *Many cases are idiopathic*

2. *Drugs and chemicals*
   Isoniazid, vincristine, amiodarone
   Lead, mercury
   Many organic chemicals

3. *Metabolic*
   Diabetes mellitus
   Amyloidosis
   Acute intermittent porphyria

4. *Deficiency states*
   B_{12} deficiency
   Alcoholism
   Beri-beri
   Pellagra

5. *Infections*
   Leprosy
   Diphtheria
   Tetanus
   Botulism

6. *Miscellaneous*
   'Acute infective polyneuritis' of Guillain-Barré
   Collagen-vascular disease, esp. polyarteritis and rheumatoid disease
   Malignancy
   Sarcoidosis

7. *Congenital*
   Rare hereditary ataxias and neuropathies

MULTIPLE SCLEROSIS

Characterized by multiple c.n.s. lesions scattered in time and place

Clinical features
1. Spastic weakness, usually starting in legs
2. Retrobulbar neuritis:
   Misty vision
   Painful eye movements
   Slightly swollen optic disc
   Central scotoma
   (Optic atrophy may develop)
3. Numbness and paraesthesiae
4. Diplopia
5. Vertigo
6. Cerebellar signs:
   Intention tremor
   Nystagmus (may be worse in the abducting eye)
   'Scanning' speech
7. Sphincter disturbance and impotence
8. Euphoria or other mental change
9. Painful flexor spasms

CAUSES OF EPILEPSY

1. **Idiopathic**

2. **Focal cerebral lesions**
   (i) Birth injury or cerebral malformation
   (ii) Tumour
   (iii) Trauma, scar, irradiation atrophy
   (iv) Vascular
      CVA
      Hypertension
      Vasculitis e.g. SLE
   (v) Infection
      Encephalitis or meningitis
      Abscess or tuberculoma
      Syphilis (GPI or gumma)
      Hydatid cysts, cysticercosis or toxoplasmosis
   (vi) Degenerative disease, e.g. presenile dementia

3. **Metabolic**
   (i) Pyrexia in children
   (ii) Anoxia, hypoglycaemia or hypocalcaemia
   (iii) Electrolyte imbalance, e.g. water intoxication
   (iv) Uraemia
   (v) Hepatic coma
   (vi) Drugs and toxins
      Lead poisoning
      Withdrawal of alcohol or barbiturates
      'Overdose' (e.g. antidepressants)

Endocrinology

THE PITUITARY

HYPOTHALAMIC CONTROL OF THE ANTERIOR PITUITARY

Stimulating hormones

1. Thyrotrophin releasing hormone (TRH)
2. Corticotrophin releasing factor (CRF)
3. Somatotrophln (GH) releasing hormone (GHRH)
4. Luteinising hormone releasing hormone (LHRH)
5. Follicle-stimulating hormone releasing hormone (FSHRH)

Inhibiting hormones
1. Prolactin inhibiting factor (PIF)
2. Melanocyte-stimulating hormone inhibiting factor (MIF)
3. Somatostatin (GH-release inhibiting hormone)

CLINICAL FEATURES OF ACROMEGALY

Symptoms
1. Often insidious, with no symptoms
2. Headaches
3. Paraesthesiae (median nerve compression)
4. Weakness and joint pains
5. Polyuria
6. Impotence and loss of libido in men
7. Hirsutism and amenorrhoea in women
8. Visual deterioration
9. Galactorrhoea

Signs
1. Characteristic facies, large hands and feet
2. Leathery furrowed skin. May be seborrhoea, hyperhidrosis or pigmentation
3. Hoarse deep voice
4. Nontoxic goitre
5. Progressive kyphosis
6. Bitemporal hemianopia, optic atrophy, ocular palsies
7. Generalized splanchnomegaly
8. Cardiac failure (hypertension and ischaemia)
9. Signs of diabetes mellitus or its complications
10. Hypopituitarism
11. Thyrotoxicosis

HYPOPITUITARISM

Causes
1. Tumours:
   (i) Eosinophil adenoma
   (ii) Chromophobe adenoma
   (iii) Craniopharyngioma
   (iv) Metastatic cancer
2. Iatrogenic — hypophysectomy or irradiation
3. Pituitary necrosis due to ante- or postpartum haemorrhage (Sheehan's syndrome)
4. Granulomatous infiltration, e.g. sarcoidosis
5. Trauma
6. Infection, e.g. TB meningitis

Clinical features
Loss of anterior pituitary hormones is usually partial, in the following order of frequency:

1. *Somatotrophin (GH):*
   (i) Dwarfism in children
   (ii) Insulin sensitivity in adults

2. *Prolactin:*
   Failure of lactation in post-partum patients

3. *Gonadotrophins:*
   (i) Delayed puberty in children
   (ii) Loss of body hair, fine wrinkled skin, impotence, infertility and amenorrhoea in adults

4. *Thyrotrophin (TSH):*
   Hypothyroidism

5. *Corticotrophin (ACTH):*
   Hypoadrenalism (asthenia, nausea, vomiting, hypoglycaemia, collapse)

6. *Melanocyte-stimulating hormone (MSH):*
   Skin pallor

CLINICAL FEATURES OF HYPOTHALAMIC LESIONS

1. Diabetes insipidus with variable deficiencies of anterior pituitary hormones
2. Obesity
3. Somnolence
4. Variations in body temperature
5. Precocious puberty
6. Irregular menstruation

THE THYROID

HYPOTHYROIDISM

Causes

(A) *Primary (Thyroid gland failure)*
1. Autoimmune thyroiditis. Hashimoto's disease and its atrophic variant, myxoedema. In Hashimoto's the thyroid is large and may be tender, but in myxoedema it is impalpable. Circulating thyroid antibodies occur in both
2. Iatrogenic:
    (i) Surgery
    (ii) Irradiation
    (iii) Antithyroid drugs

    6. Endemic goitre
    7. Subacute thyroiditis

3. Endemic cretinism (maternal iodine deficiency)
4. Absence or maldevelopment of thyroid gland (rare)
5. Dyshormonogenesis (rare congenital enzyme defects affecting hormone synthesis) *inc Pendreds syndrome*

(B) *Secondary (TSH deficiency)*
1. Pituitary lesion
2. Rarely hypothalamic lesion (due to thyrotrophin releasing hormone deficiency)

Clinical features
1. Mental and physical sluggishness
2. Cold intolerance
3. Constipation
4. Weight gain
5. Croaking voice, with slow speech
6. Rough, dry yellowish skin *Peaches & Cream complexion*
7. 'Myxoedema facies' with generalized thickening of subcutaneous tissue, periorbital puffiness, brittle sparse hair and thin eyebrows
8. Bradycardia
9. Delayed relaxation of tendon jerks

Less commonly
10. Anaemia
11. Cyanosis, Raynaud's phenomenon or angina
12. Carpal tunnel syndrome
13. Perceptive deafness
14. Myalgia or arthralgia
15. 'Myxoedema madness'
16. Coma

CAUSES OF 'NON-TOXIC' GOITRE

1. 'Simple' colloid goitre (idiopathic), common during puberty and pregnancy
2. Iodine deficiency
3. Goitrogens, e.g. antithyroid drugs, excess iodine
4. Auto-immune thyroiditis (Hashimoto's)

Possibility of malignancy is suggested by:
1. Asymmetrical enlargement with 'cold area' on scan
2. Very hard thyroid
3. Pressure effects, e.g. hoarseness
4. Cervical lymphadenopathy

HYPERTHYROIDISM

Causes
1. Graves' disease
2. Toxic multinodular goitre. Resembles Graves' disease but patients tend to be older, with fewer eye signs
3. Toxic adenoma
4. Iatrogenic (excess thyroid hormone)

Clinical features of Graves' disease

Thyroid gland
1. Goitre, usually diffuse (but may be nodular)
2. Increased thyroid vascularity (thrill, bruit)

Metabolic
3. Increased heat production (warm moist skin, heat intolerance)
4. Weight loss, increased appetite, diarrhoea
5. Tachycardia, exertional dyspnoea, hyperdynamic circulation   *Atrial Fibrillation*
6. Tiredness, irritability, nervousness
7. Fine tremor, hyperkinesia
8. Proximal muscle weakness with hyperactive reflexes
9. Occasionally, bone pain due to osteoporosis
10. In elderly patients, atrial fibrillation or cardiac failure

Extra-thyroid manifestations (possibly immunological)
11. Eye signs:
    Eyelid oedema
    Conjunctivitis
    Exophthalmos
    Lid retraction or lag
    Ophthalmoplegia (usually superior rectus)
12. Pretibial myxoedema
13. Thyroid acropachy (clubbing)
14. Vitiligo
15. Splenomegaly

Management of thyrotoxicosis

1. *Indications for thyroidectomy*
   (i) Possible malignancy
   (ii) Pressure symptoms
   (iii) Retrosternal goitre
   (iv) Large goitre
   (v) Refusal or failure of medical treatment
   (vi) Hypersensitivity to antithyroid drugs
       Cosmetic

2. *Indications for medical treatment*
   (i) Children
   (ii) Pregnancy
   (iii) Mild hyperthyroidism with small goitre
   (iv) Patients unsuitable for surgery

3. *Indications for radioiodine therapy*
   (i) Relapse after thyroidectomy
   (ii) Patients over age 45

   Subsequent hypothyroidism is common (about 40% at 10 years)

THE PARATHYROIDS

HYPERPARATHYROIDISM

Causes

1. *Primary*
   (i) Adenoma (85%)
   (ii) Hyperplasia
   (iii) Carcinoma

2. *Secondary*
   Hyperplasia due to chronic renal failure, osteomalacia or rickets

3. *Tertiary*
   A complication of secondary parathyroidism in which
   autonomous hyperparathyroidism develops

CAUSES OF HYPERCALCAEMIA
1. Endocrine
   1°, 2° + 3° Hyperparathyroidism
   Hyperthyroidism (unusual)
   Adrenocortical insufficiency (rare)
2. Metabolic disturbances
   Vit D excess
   Milk-alkali syndrome
   Sarcoidosis
3. Bone disease
   Metastatic ca, myeloma, reticuloses
   Non-metastatic bone disease
   Paget's disease - immobilised
4. Drugs
   Vit B4, thiazides, ion exchange resins

HYPOCALCAEMIA
1. Normal ionised Ca++
   1. Hypoproteinaemia - nephrotic syndr
                         hepatic cirrho
                         severe malnutrit
   2. Renal failure
2. ↓ ionised Ca++
   a. Endocrine - hypoparathyroid i
      True - Iatrogenic
             Auto-immune
             Idiopathic
      False - pseudohypoparathyr
   b. Vit D abnormalities
      - malabsorption - GI di
      anti convulsants
      renal failure
   c. Others eg. pancreatitis (

Clinical features

1. *Due to hypercalcaemia*
    (i) Anorexia, nausea and vomiting
    (ii) Constipation
    (iii) Polydipsia and polyuria
    (iv) Lethargy progressing to coma and convulsions

2. *Metastatic calcification*
    (i) Renal calculi
    (ii) Nephrocalcinosis
    (iii) Conjunctival deposits and keratopathy

3. *Bone resorption*
    (i) Pain and deformity
    (ii) Pathological fractures

4. *Rarely*
    (i) Peptic ulcer
    (ii) Pancreatitis
    (iii) Multiple endocrine adenomatosis
    (iv) Pseudo-gout (pyrophosphate arthropathy)
    (v) Zollinger-Ellison syndrome (pancreatic adenomas, gastric HCl and pepsin overproduction with recurrent gut ulceration)

HYPOPARATHYROIDISM

Causes
1. Postoperative (e.g. thyroidectomy)
2. Idiopathic (possibly autoimmune)
3. Neonatal (transient, but dangerous)

Clinical features

1. *Due to hypocalcaemia*
    (i) Tetany (paraesthesiae, stridor, cramps, hyperreflexia) Trousseau's and Chvostek's signs are present
    (ii) Convulsions (especially in children)
    (iii) Cataracts

2. *In idiopathic hypoparathyroidism*
    (i) Mental subnormality
    (ii) Dry skin, sparse hair, poor teeth, nail dystrophy often with Candidosis
    (iii) Papilloedema and calcified basal ganglia (mimics brain tumour)
    (iv) Other auto-immune disorders, e.g. hypoadrenalism, pernicious anaemia

THE ADRENALS

CUSHING'S SYNDROME

Clinical features
1. Obesity of trunk and face with 'buffalo hump'
2. Hypertension
3. Skin changes:
   (i) Striae
   (ii) Bruising
   (iii) Hirsutism
   (iv) Pigmentation

4. Osteoporosis
5. Proximal myopathy
6. Menstrual disturbances
7. Neurosis or psychosis
8. Facial plethora due to polycythaemia

Laboratory features
1. Increased plasma 11 — hydroxycorticosteroids ('cortisol')
   Normal values —

9 a.m.	12 midnight
190–690 nmol/l	80–190 nmol/l
(7–25 μg/100 ml)	(3–7 μg/100 ml)

   Loss of diurnal rhythm occurs early in Cushing's syndrome (i.e. midnight samples give increased value)
2. Polycythaemia with leucocytosis and eosinophil decrease
3. Hypokalaemia, with sodium in upper normal range
4. 'Diabetic' glucose tolerance test
5. 24 hour urinary 'free 11-hydroxycorticosteroids' increased
   Low dosage dexamethasone (0.5 mg q.d.s. for 2 days) causes little suppression in Cushing's syndrome
   High dosage dexamethasone (2 mg q.d.s. for 2 days) causes suppression in adrenal hyperplasia, but has little or no effect in adrenal adenoma or carcinoma, or ectopic ACTH secretion due to extra-adrenal carcinoma

CAUSES OF HYPOADRENALISM

Acute
1. Stress occurring patients with chronic hypoadrenalism
2. Septicaemia, especially meningococcal
3. Surgical adrenalectomy, e.g. for breast cancer

Chronic

(A) *Primary*
1. Auto-immune adrenalitis (Addison's)
2. TB
3. Metastatic cancer deposits occur commonly, but rarely cause hypoadrenalism

(B) *Secondary (ACTH deficiency)*
1. Pituitary or hypothalamic disease
2. Prolonged corticosteroid therapy

Clinical features of chronic hypoadrenalism
1. Pigmentation, especially in exposed skin, mouth, areolae, palmar creases, pressure areas and scars
2. Debility and tiredness
3. Nausea, vomiting, weight loss, abdominal pain, diarrhoea
4. Hypotension, with low-volume pulse
5. Hypoglycaemia, especially reactive after a meal
6. Loss of body hair in women
7. Depression

Laboratory features of hypoadrenalism
1. Plasma 11-hydroxycorticosteroids may be normal or low, but fail to respond adequately to 250 μg Synacthen i.m. (should rise by more than 193 nmol/l (7 μg/100 ml) at 30 minutes)
2. Low plasma sodium and chloride, with raised potassium and urea
3. Low voltage e.c.g. with flat T waves
4. Low blood sugar

DIABETES MELLITUS

Differences between the 2 main types of diabetes mellitus

'Juvenile'	*'Maturity onset'*
1. Thin	Obese
2. Young	Middle-aged or elderly
3. Tendency to ketosis	Resistant to ketosis
4. Low insulin secretion	Normal or increased insulin secretion
5. Sensitive to insulin	Insulin resistant
6. Require treatment with insulin	Respond to diet, and oral hypoglycaemic drugs

Differences between 'diabetic' and hypoglycaemic coma

Ketoacidaemic coma	*Hypoglycaemic coma*
1. Preceded by infection or insulin underdosage	Preceded by exercise, missed meal or insulin overdosage
2. Onset over hours or days	Onset in minutes
3. Deep rapid breathing	Stertorous breathing
4. Dehydration	Normal hydration
5. Sweating absent	Sweating marked
6. C.n.s. changes unusual	C.n.s. changes common, especially Babinski response
7. Urine — usually glycosuria and ketonuria	Urine not helpful

Complications of diabetes mellitus

1. *Ocular*
   (i) Blurred vision due to fluctuations in blood sugar
   (ii) Cataracts
   (iii) Retinopathy:
      a. Venous engorgement
      b. Capillary microaneurysms
      c. 'Blot' haemorrhages
      d. 'Waxy' exudates
      e. Retinitis proliferans (new vessel formation)
      f. Retinal detachment
      g. Vitreous haemorrhage and fibrosis
   (iv) Rubeosis iridis (new blood vessels over iris) — may cause glaucoma
2. *Neurological*
   (i) Peripheral neuropathy (early sign is loss of ankle jerks and malleolar vibration sense)
   (ii) Mononeuritis multiplex (neuropathy of several peripheral or cranial nerves; often asymmetrical)
   (iii) Autonomic neuropathy:
      a. Diarrhoea
      b. Postural hypotension
      c. Impotence
      d. Abnormal sweating
      e. Dependent oedema

3. *Renal*
   (i) Pyelonephritis, sometimes with papillary necrosis
   (ii) Glomerulonephritis
      a. Kimmelstiel — Wilson (eosinophilic nodules in glomerular tuft)
      b. Proliferative, with sclerosed basement membrane
   (iii) Atherosclerosis and hypertensive vascular changes

4. *Vascular*
   Occlusion by atheroma (large vessels) or endarteritis (small vessels) may cause ischaemia of feet, myocardium, brain or kidneys

5. *Dermatological*
   (i) Fat atrophy or hypertrophy at insulin injection sites
   (ii) Ulcers due to neuropathy or ischaemia
   (iii) Infections, especially furuncles and Candidosis
   (iv) Pigmented scars over shins ('diabetic dermopathy')
   (v) Xanthomata
   (vi) Necrobiosis lipoidica

6. *Systemic infections*
   Incidence of TB and deep mycoses is increased

CAUSES OF DWARFISM

1. **'Constitutional'**
   Racial, familial or sporadic

2. **Nutritional**
   (i) Starvation
   (ii) Malabsorption
   (iii) Protein loss

3. **Chromosomal defects**
   (i) Trisomies, e.g. Down's
   (ii) Turner's

4. **Skeletal defects**
   (i) Rickets
   (ii) Achondroplasia
   (iii) Gargoylism (Hurler's)

5. **Chronic systemic disease**
   (i) Cyanotic congenital heart disease
   (ii) Renal failure
   (iii) Hepatic failure
   (iv) Pulmonary disease
   (v) Anaemia
   (vi) Infections, e.g. TB
   (vii) Long-term steroid therapy (e.g. for asthma)

6. **Endocrine disease**
   (i) Sexual precocity
   (ii) Hypopituitarism
   (iii) Hypothyroidism
   (iv) Congenital adrenal hyperplasia

7. **Miscellaneous rare diseases**
   Diseases of unknown cause, e.g. progeria

CAUSES OF GYNAECOMASTIA

1. Neonatal, or normal puberty
2. Cirrhosis
3. Malignancy
4. Testicular or adrenal tumours
5. Drugs
    (i) Oestrogens
    (ii) Cyproterone acetate
    (iii) Spironolactone
    (iv) Cimetidine
    (v) Methyldopa
    (vi) Digoxin
6. Klinefelter's syndrome (XXY)

CAUSES OF GALACTORRHOEA

1. Physiological (postpartum or neonatal)
2. Prolactin-secreting pituitary tumour
3. Ectopic prolactin, e.g. bronchial ca
4. Drugs
    (i) Phenothiazines
    (ii) Oral contraceptives
    (iii) Methyldopa

ORAL CONTRACEPTIVES

Regimes

1. Oestrogen (mestranol or ethinyloestradiol) and progestogen in combination for cycles of 20 to 22 days
2. Oestrogen alone for 15 days, followed by a combination tablet for 7 days
3. Progestogen alone, daily without interruption

Side-effects of oral contraceptives
1. *Symptoms due to oestrogens*
   Fluid retention, weight gain
   Nausea and vomiting
   Headache
   Tiredness and irritability
   Venous hypertension in legs
   Increased menstrual loss

2. *Symptoms due to progestogens*
   Depression
   Acne
   Decreased libido, dry vagina
   Muscle cramps
   Breast discomfort
   Reduced menstrual loss

3. *Gynaecological*
   Amenorrhoea on contraceptive withdrawal
   Cervical erosion
   Vaginal Candidosis
   Increase in size of fibroids

4. *Endocrine and metabolic*
   Abnormal carbohydrate tolerance
   Increased plasma triglycerides and cholesterol
   Abnormal liver function tests (including BSP)
   Plasma protein changes, e.g. increased transferrin
   Increased serum PBI, thyroxine and plasma cortisol
   Rarely — Hypertension
               Chloasma
               Galactorrhoea
               Gall-stones

5. *Thromboembolic effects*
   Increased risk of thrombosis (e.g. coronary, cerebral) or
   embolism (e.g. pulmonary) due to increased clotting factors and
   platelet stickiness

Contra-indications to oestrogenic oral contraceptives
1. Pregnancy
2. Hepatic disease
3. Breast or cervical carcinoma
4. History of thrombosis or embolism
5. Care is required in patients with a history of epilepsy,
   hypertension, varicose veins, oedema, diabetes mellitus,
   migraine or fibroids. Women over age 35 are at increased risk of
   thromboembolic disease (esp. smokers)

OSTEOPOROSIS

A reduction in bone mass below the normal expected for the age and sex of the patient. Histologically the trabecular bone is reduced, and the mineral-matrix ratio is approximately normal

Common causes
1. Old age
2. Immobilization
3. Glucocorticoid therapy (or Cushing's disease)
4. Sex hormone deficiency, e.g. premature menopause, Turner's syndrome
5. Rheumatoid arthritis causes localized osteoporosis

OSTEOMALACIA

A reduction in the mineral-matrix ratio, although the total bone mass may be normal, decreased or even increased

Causes
1. Deficiency of cholecalciferol (vitamin D)
    (i) Inadequate diet, possibly aggravated by pregnancy or lack of u.v. radiation
    (ii) Malabsorption
    (iii) Anticonvulsants
2. Chronic renal failure
3. Hepatic disease (disturbed vitamin D metabolism)

PAGET'S DISEASE
Clinical features

1. Often asymptomatic. Incidence increases with age
2. Bone deformity
    (i) Enlarged skull
    (ii) Sabre tibia
    (iii) Long bone fractures
3. Nerve entrapment,
    (i) Deafness
    (ii) Basilar invagination
    (iii) Cervical spondylosis
4. High output cardiac failure
5. Increased incidence of bone sarcoma

Renal disease

Classical presentations of renal disease

1. Haematuria alone
2. Proteinuria alone
3. Nephrotic syndrome (severe proteinuria, hypoalbuminaemia and peripheral oedema).
4. Nephritic syndrome (haematuria, hypertension and peripheral oedema).
5. Acute renal failure (oliguria with acute uraemia)
6. Chronic renal failure (polyuria with insidious uraemia)

Renal disease which affects the glomeruli is called glomerulonephritis, and this is classified by the pathology shown on renal biopsy. Many diseases can cause more than one of the above presentations. Thus membranous glomerulonephritis usually causes the nephrotic syndrome, but it can occasionally present as acute or chronic renal failure.

RENAL FAILURE
CAUSES OF ACUTE RENAL FAILURE

(A) Prerenal

1. Loss of blood, plasma or water and electrolytes
2. Hypotension with normal blood volume, e.g. myocardial infarct or septicaemic shock

(B) Renal
1. Acute-on-chronic failure, precipitated by renal infection or dehydration
2. Acute tubular necrosis' (or rarely cortical necrosis)
    (i) Sustained hypotension
    (ii) Obstetric causes, e.g. abortion or ante-partum haemorrhage
    (iii) Septicaemia (especially Gram-negative)
    (iv) Free circulating haemoglobin
    (v) Extensive tissue damage
    (vi) Toxins, e.g. heavy metals, carbon tetrachloride
3. Primary renal disease
    (i) Acute glomerulonephritis
    (ii) Fulminating pyelonephritis
    (iii) Acute 'collagen vascular disease'
4. Hepato-renal syndromes (including Weil's disease)

(C) Postrenal
Obstruction in urinary tract (p. 127)

CAUSES OF CHRONIC RENAL FAILURE

1. Glomerulonephritis
2. Pyelonephritis or TB
3. Hypertension
4. Collagen vascular disease, especially SLE and PN
5. Metabolic
    (i) Diabetes mellitus
    (ii) Gout
    (iii) Chronic potassium depletion
    (iv) Chronic analgesic ingestion
    (v) Amyloidosis
6. Obstruction in renal tract
7. Congenital
    (i) Polycystic kidney
    (ii) Tubular acidosis
    (iii) Fanconi syndrome

CLINICAL FEATURES OF SEVERE 'URAEMIA'

1. **Dermatological**
   (i) Pruritus
   (ii) Pallor
   (iii) Pigmentation
   (iv) Petechiae
   (v) Rarely 'urea frost'

2. **Neurological**
   (i) Mental changes (confusion, paranoia, etc.)
   (ii) Apathy and weakness
   (iii) Muscle twitching
   (iv) Coma in terminal cases
   (v) Peripheral neuropathy in chronic undialysed cases

3. **Cardiovascular**
   (i) Pericarditis
   (ii) Cardiac failure due to salt and water overload
   (iii) Hypertension
   (iv) Arrhythmia (due to hyperkalaemia)

4. **Gastrointestinal**
   (i) Dry mouth, foetor, may be parotitis
   (ii) Anorexia, nausea and vomiting
   (iii) Hiccups
   (iv) GI tract ulceration and bleeding

5. **Genitourinary**
   (i) In acute renal failure — oliguria (<300 ml/24 hr)
   (ii) In chronic renal failure — polyuria with fixed urinary specific gravity (1.010)

6. **Respiratory**
   Hyperventilation due to acidosis

7. **Haematological**
   (i) Anaemia due to:
       GI bleeding
       Haemolysis
       Dietary restrictions
       Erythropoietin deficiency
   (i) Bleeding tendency due to platelet dysfunction
   (iii) Susceptibility to secondary infection

(continued)

8. **Defects in bone and calcium metabolism**
   (i) Osteomalacia ('renal rickets' in children)
   (ii) Secondary or tertiary hyperparathyroidism (osteitis fibrosa cystica)
   (iii) Patchy osteosclerosis
   (iv) Occasionally osteoporosis
   (v) Occasionally metastatic calcification of muscles, blood-vessels and conjunctivae

FACTORS WHICH MAY PRECIPITATE 'URAEMIA'

1. Fluid and electrolyte imbalance
2. Infection, systemic or urinary
3. Increased protein ingestion
4. Obstruction of renal tract
5. Catabolic or nephrotoxic drugs (e.g. tetracycline)
6. Congestive cardiac failure
7. Gastrointestinal haemorrhage or surgery

CLASSIFICATION OF GLOMERULONEPHRITIS

1. **Focal glomerulonephritis**
   Increased cell proliferation affecting only *some* parts of *some* glomeruli
   Occurs commonly as a primary disease but also occurs secondary to embolic nephritis (bacterial endocarditis), polyarteritis nodosa, and Henoch-Schönlein purpura

2. **Proliferative**
   (Usually secondary to Group A Streptococcal infection)
   All glomeruli are affected, with swelling and increased number of cells. 'Crescents' occur, especially in subacute cases
   Electron microscopy shows deposits on the capillary basement membrane

3. **Membranous**
   Uniform thickening of capillary basement membrane
   Tubules may contain lipid

4. **Minimal lesion**
   No change on light microscopy, but there may be lipid in the proximal tubules
   Electron microscopy shows fusion of foot processes of the glomerular epithelium

   N.B. Immunofluorescent tests are also helpful

CAUSES OF NEPHROTIC SYNDROME

1. Glomerulonephritis accounts for 80% (usually membranous in adults)
2. Metabolic
   (i) Diabetes mellitus
   (ii) Amyloidosis
   (iii) Myelomatosis
3. SLE
4. Drugs — mercurials, penicillamine, troxidone

N.B. Malaria is an important cause in endemic areas

CAUSES OF ACUTE NEPHROTIC SYNDROME

Mainly the various types of proliferative glomerulonephritis (incl. polyarteritis nodosa, SLE and Henoch-Schönlein purpura) but almost any renal disease can occasionally present with this syndrome

Causes of Nephrotic Syndrome ⟨ Proteinuria
                                Hypoproteinaemia
                                Oedema.

1. Minimal lesion GMN
2. Membranous GMN
3. Mesangiocapillary GMN
4. Amyloid – 1°
              2°
5. Renal vein thrombosis
6. Diabetic nephropathy
7. Drugs – penicillamine
                gold
8. SLE , PAN
9. Tumours
10. P. malariae.

TYPES OF RENAL TUBULAR DYSFUNCTION

1. **Renal disease affecting medulla,** e.g. pyelonephritis
   Impairment of urinary concentration, acidification and electrolyte reabsorption

2. **Renal glycosuria**

3. **'Vitamin D resistant rickets'**
   Inability to reabsorb phosphate

4. **Idiopathic hypercalcuria**
   Inability to reabsorb calcium

5. **Renal tubular acidosis**
   Inability to acidify the urine causes metabolic acidosis. Less calcium is bound to protein and calcium filtration is increased, leading to nephrocalcinosis and renal stones

6. **Cystinuria**
   Defect in reabsorption of cystine, lysine, ornithine and arginine

7. **Fanconi syndrome** (defect of proximal tubular function due to one of many possible causes)
   Defective reabsorption of glucose, phosphate and amino-acids. Usually proteinuria, with inability to concentrate or acidify urine. Adult cases may be due to renal toxins (e.g. mercury, stored tetracycline)
   Childhood cases are associated with cystinosis

8. **Nephrogenic diabetes insipidus**
   Impaired response to ADH

CLINICAL FEATURES OF POTASSIUM DEPLETION

1. Muscle weakness
2. Apathy, anorexia and confusion
3. Ileus
4. Increased cardiac excitability and digitalis toxicity
5. Thirst and polyuria
6. Renal lesions
   (i) Fanconi syndrome (q.v.)
   (ii) In severe prolonged depletion, interstitial inflammation and fibrosis occur

CAUSES OF POLYURIA

1. Chronic renal failure
2. Diabetes mellitus
3. Compulsive water drinking
4. Diabetes insipidus
    (i) Pituitary (deficiency of ADH)
    (ii) Nephrogenic (no response to ADH)
5. Potassium depletion
6. Hypercalcaemia

CAUSES OF PROTEINURIA

1. Contamination (semen, prostatic or vaginal secretion)
2. Postural (orthostatic)
3. Renal disease
    (i)   Glomerulonephritis, especially nephrotic syndrome
    (ii) Pyelonephritis
    (iii) Obstructive nephropathy
    (iv) Malignant hypertension
    (v)   Tuberculosis   Amyloid
4. Disease of renal tract, e.g. cystitis
5. May be slight albuminuria in fever or congestive heart failure
6. Multiple myeloma (Bence-Jones protein)

CAUSES OF HAEMATURIA

(A) Kidney lesions
1. Glomerulonephritis, pyelonephritis, TB
2. Trauma
3. Anticoagulant overdose, bleeding diathesis
4. Hypernephroma
5. Renal infarct (including polyarteritis nodosa)
6. Bacterial endocarditis

(B) Renal tract lesions
1. Papillary tumour of bladder
2. Acute cystitis (including cyclophosphamide toxicity)
3. Calculi
4. Prostatic lesions:
    Hypertrophy
    Cancer
    Prostatitis
5. Urethral inflammation or trauma
6. TB (now rare)

✓ CAUSES OF URINARY TRACT OBSTRUCTION

1. Stone
2. Stricture (post-op or inflammatory)   ⎫
3. Stenosis (congenital)   ⎬ occur throughout
4. Neoplasm   ⎭ the urinary tract
5. Clot
6. Neuromuscular incoordination   ⎫
7. Retroperitoneal fibrosis   ⎬ ureter
8. Spread of cancer from pelvic organs   ⎭
9. Prostatic enlargement or cancer   ⎫
10. Retroverted gravid uterus   ⎬ bladder neck
11. Trauma of labour   ⎭
12. Congenital valves   ⎫ urethra
13. Phimosis or paraphimosis   ⎭

Common causes of acute retention in adults are:
Males   *Females*
1. Post-operative retention   1. Trauma of labour
2. Prostatic lesions   2. Pressure from uterus
                                  (fetus or fibroid)
3. Urethral stricture   3. Hysteria

Remember that retention may also be due to a neurological llesion such as DS, tabes or cord compression

URINARY CALCULI

FACTORS WHICH PREDISPOSE TO URINARY CALCULI

1. Metabolic abnormalities (q.v.)
2. Urinary tract infections
3. Urinary tract stasis
4. Foreign bodies in urinary tract
5. Geographical factors (e.g. hot climate, hard water)

METABOLIC CAUSES OF URINARY CALCULI

Calcium stones
1. Hypercalcuria (on normal diet, >300 mg/24 hr in male or >250 mg/24 hr in female)
     (i) Idiopathic hypercalcuria
    (ii) Hyperparathyroidism
   (iii) Vitamin D excess
   (iv) Sarcoidosis
    (v) Milk alkali syndrome
   (vi) Renal tubular acidosis
  (vii) Malignancy
 (viii) Immobilization
   (ix) Cushing's syndrome
2. Alkaline urine
3. Oxaluria

Uric acid stones
Primary or secondary gout
Uricosuric drugs

Cystine stones
Cystinuria
Fanconi syndrome with cystinosis

Xanthine stones
Xanthinuria

NEUROLOGICAL CONTROL OF BLADDER FUNCTION

Normal bladder capacity is 300–400 ml and larger volumes should stimulate the desire to micturate. Afferent fibres travel via parasympathetic nerves to spinal 'micturition centre' (S 2, 3, 4) and bladder contraction is initiated by parasympathetic efferents. The spinal 'micturition centre' is normally inhibited by higher motor centres, which bombard it with facilitatory impulses when micturition begins, so that the bladder empties completely

TYPES OF DYSFUNCTION

1. **Lack of normal inhibition**
    Frequency with small volumes
    Occurs in anxiety, cold weather, etc.

2. **Atonic bladder**
    Distended bladder with overflow, but no desire to micturate
    Occurs with sensory neuropathy, e.g. diabetes mellitus, tabes dorsalis

3. **Automatic bladder**
    Bladder empties partially when volume of about 250 ml is reached, but without desire to micturate
    Occurs with cord section above S 2, 3, 4

4. **Autonomous bladder**
    Large residual urine volume, with weak uncoordinated bladder contractions but no desire to micturate. Occurs with LMN cord lesions at S 2, 3, 4 level
    Unilateral neurological lesions may cause either frequency with small volumes or a large hypotonic bladder with residual urine after micturition

RENAL CLEARANCE

The number of ml of plasma which contains the amount of a substance excreted in the urine in one minute is the renal clearance of that substance, i.e. $C = UV/PT$ ml
where U = concentration of substance in urine
$\quad\quad V$ = volume of urine collected in time T
$\quad\quad P$ = concentration of substance in plasma

Rheumatology

PATTERNS OF POLYARTHROPATHY

Primary osteoarthrosis
Symmetrical, affecting many joints
1. Knees
2. Great toes and thumbs: MP joints
3. Fingers: terminal IP joints
4. Acromioclavicular joints
5. Small joints of spine

Secondary osteoarthrosis
Asymmetrical, affecting weight-bearing joints
1. Knee
2. Hip
3. Intervertebral discs

Rheumatoid arthritis
1. Hands: intercarpal joints, MP joints and proximal IP joints
2. Feet: tarsal and lateral MP joints
3. Knees
4. Small joints of cervical spine and subacromial bursae

Ankylosing spondylitis
1. Spine and both sacro-iliac joints
2. Knees, shoulders, wrists

Psoriasis
1. Hands, terminal IP joints
2. Sacroiliac joints
3. 'Rheumatoid' pattern

Reiter's
1. Ankles and all joints of feet
2. Knees
3. Hips, sacroiliac joint and spine

JOINT COMPLICATIONS OF RHEUMATOID ARTHRITIS

1. Deformity, subluxation, misalignment, swelling
2. Infection
3. Tendon rupture
4. Synovial sac protrusion and rupture (e.g. Baker's cyst)
5. Hoarseness due to cricoarytenoid arthritis
6. Deafness due to auditory ossicle arthritis
7. Juxta-articular osteoporosis
8. Muscle atrophy secondary to disuse

EXTRA-ARTICULAR MANIFESTATIONS OF RHEUMATOID DISEASE

1. Anaemia
   (i) Fe deficiency (GI blood loss caused by drugs)
   (ii) Defective iron utilization (anaemia of chronic disorders)
   (iii) Marrow depression
2. Pulmonary
   (i) Pleuritis, effusions
   (ii) Nodules in lung or pleura
   (iii) Fibrosing alveolitis
3. Cardias
   (i) Pericarditis
   (ii) Nodules in myocardium
4. Ocular
   (i) Scleritis, episcleritis
   (ii) Scleromalacia perforans
   (iii) Sicca syndrome (Sjögren's)
5. Arteritis
   (i) Digital ischaemia (may be Raynand's)
   (ii) Nail fold lesions
   (iii) Leg ulcers
   (iv) Mesenteric ischaemia
6. Peripheral neuropathy (due to vasculitis)
7. Entrapment neuropathy, e.g. spinal cord at cervical level, or carpal tunnel syndrome
8. Felty's syndrome (R.A. with leucopenia and splenomegaly)
9. Lymphadenopathy
10. Amyloidosis

CAUSES OF A SINGLE HOT RED JOINT

1. Traumatic, e.g. sprained ankle
2. Septic arthritis
   May be secondary to penetrating injury, osteomyelitis, septicaemia, rheumatoid arthritis or osteoarthrosis
3. Gout or pseudo-gout (chondrocalcinosis or periarticular calcification)
4. Haemophilia
5. Gonococcal arthritis
6. Occasionally rheumatoid arthritis

CAUSES OF A TRANSIENT 'FLITTING' ARTHRITIS

1. Rheumatic fever
2. Henoch-Schönlein purpura
3. Serum sickness and drug reactions
4. SLE
5. Systemic infections
   (i) Bacterial endocarditis
   (ii) Rubella
   (iii) Infectious mononucleosis
   (iv) Infective hepatitis
   (v) Mycoplasma pneumonia
   (vi) Gonococcal or meningococcal septicaemia
6. Reiter's disease
7. Occasionally, acute rheumatoid arthritis

CLINICAL FEATURES OF POLYARTERITIS NODOSA

Usually young or middle-aged men
1. Fever, malaise, weight-loss
2. Gastrointestinal ischaemia:
   central abdominal pain
   bleeding
3. Proteinuria and haematuria. Hypertension is common
4. Peripheral neuropathy, often painful
   Focal c.n.s. lesions
5. Arthralgia and myalgia
6. Myocardial ischaemia
7. Skin lesions:
   nodules
   livedo reticularis
   necrosis and ulceration

N.B. Asthma, haemoptysis and pneumonitis may occur in association with eosinophilia and systemic vasculitis, but some authors regard this 'pulmonary' form as an entity distinct from polyarteritis nodosa.

CLINICAL FEATURES OF SYSTEMIC LUPUS ERYTHEMATOSUS

Usually young or middle-aged women
1. Fever, malaise, weight-loss
2. Arthralgia, flitting or episodic
3. Skin changes
    (i) Rash, classically in butterfly distribution. May be erythematous, urticated or purpuric
    (ii) Alopecia
    (iii) Dilated nail fold capillaries
    (iv) Raynaud's phenomenon
4. Proteinuria, glomerulonephritis, nephrotic syndrome or hypertension
5. Lymphadenopathy
6. Myocarditis, endocarditis (Libman-Sacks), or pericarditis
7. Pleurisy with effusion, pneumonitis
8. Hepatomegaly and splenomegaly
9. Pancytopenia. May be haemolysis
10. Psychosis, neuropathy or epilepsy. May be retinal exudates
11. Gastrointestinal upsets (nausea, pain, diarrhoea, etc.)

RAYNAUD'S PHENOMENON

Paroxysmal digital ischaemia, which usually causes a characteristic sequence of colour changes (white, then blue, then red)

Causes

1. *Reflex vasoconstriction*
    (i) Raynaud's disease (idiopathic)
    (ii) Vibrating machinery

2. *Arterial occlusion*
    (i) Thoracic outlet syndromes
    (ii) Atheroma. Buerger's disease

3. *Collagen-vascular diesase*, especially systemic sclerosis and SLE

4. *Increased blood viscosity*
    (i) Dysproteinaemias (macro- and cryoglobulinaemias)
    (ii) Polycythaemia, leukaemia

5. *Neurological disease*, especially syringomyelia or paralysis

Dermatology

SKIN CHANGES ASSOCIATED WITH SYSTEMIC MALIGNANCY

1. **Genetic syndromes predisposing to malignancy**
   e.g. neurofibromatosis (may develop glioma), familial tylosis (palmar keratoderma) with oesophageal caricinoma.

2. **Signs of exposure to a carcinogen**
   e.g.:
   (i) Nicotine staining of fingers
   (ii) Palmar keratoses due to arsenic

3. **Direct involvement of skin by malignant cells**
   (i) Direct spread from underlying cancer (especially breast)
   (ii) Cutaneous metastases
   (iii) Leukaemic or lymphomatous infiltrate

4. **Miscellaneous endocrine, metabolic and immunological effects**
   (i) Pigmentation, pallor or pruritus
   (ii) Acanthosis nigricans
   (iii) Dermatomyositis
   (iv) Clubbing
   (v) Widespread viral infection (e.g. herpes) due to immune paresis, etc

ECZEMA

Eczema is a distinctive inflammatory response of the skin, characterized histologically by spongiosis (epidermal oedema) and clinically by clustered papulo-vesicles with erythema and scaling.
   Many cases have a multifactorial aetiology

TYPES OF ECZEMA

(A) Exogenous
1. Primary irritant dermatitis, e.g. due to caustics, detergents or solvents
2. Allergic contact dermatitis, e.g. due to hypersensitivity to metals, rubber, medicaments, etc.
3. Infective dermatitis, e.g. around infected wounds or ulcers

(B) Endogenous
1. Atopic dermatitis (infantile eczema)
2. Seborrhoeic dermatitis
3. Discoid eczema
4. Pompholyx — vesicles on palms or soles
5. Pityriasis alba — patches of scaly eczema which leave depigmented areas
6. Asteatotic eczema — due to excessive drying ('chapping')
7. Gravitational eczema — secondary to venous insufficiency

BLISTERING ERUPTIONS

Common
1. Viral
    (i) Herpes simplex
    (ii) Herpes zoster — varicella
2. Impetigo
3. Scabies
4. Insect bites and papular urticaria
5. Bullous eczema and pompholyx
6. Drugs, e.g. barbiturate overdose, photosensitivity

Uncommon
7. Erytherma multiforme
8. Dermatitis herpetiformis
9. Pemphigoid   sub-epidermal
10. Porphyria cutanea tarda
11. Pemphigus group   intra-epidermal

Rare
12. Congenital
    (i) Epidermolysis bullosa
    (ii) Ichthyosiform erythroderma
    (iii) Incontinentia pigmenti

CAUSES OF PHOTOSENSITIVITY (ENHANCED RESPONSE TO UV IRRADIATION)

1. Drugs, e.g. phenothiazines, chlorpropamide, nalidixic acid
2. Contact photosensitizers, e.g. tar, perfumes, soaps, etc
3. Dermatoses, e.g. porphyria, polymorphic light eruption, lupus erythematosus
4. Decreased melanin in skin, e.g. albinism, vitiligo

CAUSES OF LEG ULCERS

1. Venous hypertension, with peri-capillary fibrin deposition
2. Ischaemia
    (i) Atheroma
    (ii) Arteritis
3. Neuropathy
    (i) Diabetes mellitus
    (ii) Spina bifida
    (iii) Tabes dorsalis
    (iv) Leprosy (in endemic areas)
4. Rheumatoid arthritis — ulceration is multifactorial
5. Malignancy — usually squamous-cell skin carcinoma
6. Haemolytic anaemia, especially sickle-cell
7. Gumma
8. Necrobiosis lipoidica (may be diabetic)
9. Pyoderma gangrenosum — often due to ulcerative colitis

Many leg ulcers have a multifactorial aetiology, e.g. ischaemia, anaemia, venous hypertension and infection

CAUSES OF ALOPECIA

1. Male-pattern baldness
2. Idiopathic diffuse alopecia of women — usually post-menopausal
3. 'Telogen effluvium' — loss of club hairs after febrile illness, surgery or parturition
4. Alopecia areata
5. Drugs:
   (i) Cytotoxic agents
   (ii) Anticoagulants
   (iii) Dextran
   (iv) Oral contraceptives
6. Scalp infection:
   (i) Fungi
   (ii) Pyogenic bacteria
7. Systemic disease:
   (i) Syphilis
   (ii) Hypothyroidism
   (iii) Fe deficiency
8. Traumatic:
   (i) Traction from rollers
   (ii) Scalping injury
   (iii) Burns
   (iv) Excessive bleaching, perming, etc.
9. Dermatoses:
   (i) Psoriasis
   (ii) Discoid lupus erythematosus
   (iii) Lichen planus
10. Congenital — many rare diseases, e.g. monilethrix

CAUSES OF HIRSUTISM

1. Idiopathic (including racial and familial variation)
2. Ovarian disease
   (i) Polycystic ovaries (common)
   (ii) Virilizing tumour (rare)
3. Adrenal hyperplasia or tumour
4. Androgenic drugs, e.g. methyltestosterone, anabolic steroids

CAUSES OF DIFFUSE HYPERPIGMENTATION

1. Congenital (racial or familial)
2. Irradiation, esp. u.v.r.
3. Post-inflammatory, e.g. after erythroderma
4. Endocrine causes
   (i) Pregnancy, oestrogens
   (ii) Hypoadrenalism (due to beta-lipotrophin)
   (iii) Acromegaly
5. Miscellaneous systemic diseases
   (i) Cachexia (esp. TB or malignancy)
   (ii) Chronic renal failure
   (iii) Primary biliary cirrhosis
   (iv) Haemochromatosis
   (v) Malabsorption
6. Drugs, e.g. busulphan, chlorpromazine, ACTH, arsenic

SYSTEMIC CAUSES OF GENERALIZED PRURITUS

1. Obstructive jaundice (especially biliary cirrhosis)
2. Chronic renal failure
3. Lymphoma (especially Hodgkin's) or myeloproliferative disease
   (especially polycythaemia vera)
4. Carcinoma (especially bronchial)
5. Iron deficiency
6. Hypo- or hyperthyroidism
7. Drugs
   (i) Allergy
   (ii) Pharmacological e.g. cocaine, morphine

N.B. a. Many women develop pruritus during pregnancy
     b. Scabies is easily missed in hygienic patients — Remember
        to look for burrows in the fingerwebs, and examine the
        nipples or penis for typical papules.

Causes of white patches on the skin
1. *Congenital* (rare), e.g. tuberous sclerosis, partial albinism
2. *Post-inflammatory*, e.g. eczema, burns, discoid lupus
   erythematosus
3. *Infection*, e.g. leprosy, pityriasis versicolor
4. *Immunological*, e.g. vitiligo, halo naevus

Common causes of a pigmented papule
1. Basal cell papilloma ('seborrhoeic wart')
2. Melanocytic naevus ('mole')
3. Malignant melanoma
4. Pigmented basal cell carcinoma
5. Dermatofibroma

Causes of palmar erythema
1. Dermatoses e,g. eczema or psoriasis
2. Increased oestrogens
   (i) Pregnancy
   (ii) Alcoholic cirrhosis
3. Rheumatoid arthritis
4. Shoulder-hand syndrome
5. Polycythaemia

Some causes of a circumscribed patch of red scaly rash
1. Psoriasis
2. Eczema
3. Fixed drug eruption
4. Fungus
5. Lichen simplex
6. Bowen's disease (squamous Ca-in-situ)
7. Discoid lupus erythematosus
8. Lupus vulgaris

Some causes of widespread patches of red scaly rash
1. Psoriasis
2. Eczema
3. Pityriasis rosea
4. Pityriasis versicolor
5. Secondary syphilis
6. Lichen planus
7. Fungus

Causes of erythema nodosum
1. Sarcoidosis
2. Streptococcal infection
3. TB
4. Sulphonamides
5. Ulcerative colitis or Crohn's disease
6. Other infections, e.g.
   (i) Leprosy
   (ii) Systemic mycoses
   (iii) Toxoplasmosis
   (iv) Lymphogranuloma venereum

E. nodosum.
Sarcoid
Streptococci
TB
Sulphonamides
U.C. + Crohn's
Infx - leprosy
mycoses
toxoplasmosis
lymphogranuloma
venereum

PSORIASIS

Distinctive morphological types
1. Nummular — discoid plagues, which may be confluent
2. Guttate — 'showers' of small lesions, often post-streptococcal
3. Erythrodermic — very widespread erythema, with exfoliation
4. Generalized pustular psoriasis
5. Pustular eruptions of the hands and feet
   Atypical forms are common, e.g. follicular, intertriginous, etc

   '*Napkin psoriasis*' (Psoriasiform lesions in infants) may be related
to candida infection

PATTERNS OF DRUG ERUPTIONS

Any drug can occasionally cause an eruption. Any eruption can
occasionally be mimicked by a drug reaction. The following list is far
from comprehensive:
1. Exanthemata (morbilliform etc.) e.g. penicillin
2. Urticaria e.g. penicillin
3. Erythroderma e.g. gold
4. Bullous, including erythema multiforme, e.g. sulphonamides
5. Erythema nodosum, e.g. sulphonamides
6. Purpura (due to either thrombocytopenia or vasculitis)
7. Photosensitivity e.g. chlorpromazine
8. Acneiform e.g. iodides

CAUSES OF MOUTH ULCERS

1. Aphthous ulcers
   (i) Minor
   (ii) Major
   (iii) Herpetiform
2. Squamous carcinoma (often missed)
3. Infection, e.g. herpex simplex
4. Lichen planus
5. Pemphigus or benign mucous membrane pemphigoid
6. Drugs, e.g. methotrexate
7. Trauma, e.g. from dentures
8. Behçet's, Reiter's or Stevens-Johnson (p. 141)

Three systemic diseases which cause conjunctivitis with ulcers of the mouth and genitalia:

1. **Reiter's syndrome**

   Clinical features
   (i) Non-specific urethritis, haematuria, sterile pyuria
   (ii) Recurrent conjunctivitis or uveitis
   (iii) Symmetrical subacute arthritis, tenosynovitis, periostitis
   (iv) Circinate balanitis
   (v) Buccal ulcers
   (vi) Keratoderma blenorrhagica (resembles pustular psoriasis)

2. **Stevens-Johnson syndrome**

   Clinical features
   (i) Constitutional symptoms and high fever
   (ii) Conjunctivitis, corneal ulcers, uveitis
   (iii) Oral bullae and haemorrhagic crusting
   (iv) Erythema multiforms
   (v) Urethritis, balanitis, vulvo-vaginitis
   (vi) Bronchitis, pneumonitis, or renal lesions

Behçet's syndrome

   Clinical features
   (i) Buccal ulcers with a red areola
   (ii) Conjunctivitis or uveitis
   (iii) Cutaneous pustules, dermal nodules
   (iv) Genital ulcers
   (v) C.n.s. lesions: meningo-encephalitis, brain-stem syndromes
   (vi) Thrombophlebitis *a DVT associated*

Types of porphyria
1. *Acute intermittent porphyria.* Classical triad of dark urine, abdominal pain, (sometimes with nausea or constipation) and neurophyschiatric symptoms. No skin involvement.
2. *Porphyria cutanea tarda.* Photosensitivity and skin fragility. Usually develops in middle-aged patients with hepatic disease, especially alcoholic men. Associated with increased iron stores, and treated by venesection.
3. *Erythropoietic proto-porphyria.* Photosensitivity, often starting in early life, and causing superficial linear scars on the face.

Management of medical emergencies

UNEXPECTED CARDIAC ARREST

Immediately call the 'cardiac arrest team' and give a sharp thump on the praecordium. Clear the airway, start artificial respiration (mouth-to-mouth or Ambu bag) and external cardiac compression. If the bed is sprung, move the patient to the floor.

When help arrives, arrange intubation and artificial ventilation with oxygen, and obtain an e.c.g. Start on i.v. infusion and give 100 mEq of sodium bicarbonate.

If ventricular fibrillation

1. *Defibrillate* Use 200 joules. If no response repeat with increase in output
2. Fine fibrillation (feeble low voltage) may coarsen with 1 ml. i.v. of 1/1000 adrenaline, then respond to cardioversion
3. If v.f. persists or relapses, try lignocaine 100 mg. i.v.

If asystole
1. Give 1 ml. of 1/1000 adrenaline i.v.
2. Give 5-10 ml. of 10% calcium chloride
3. Repeat if no response
4. Consider temporary pacing

Arterial pH must be corrected under laboratory control, and mannitol infusion or dexamethasone may be required for cerebral oedema.

MYOCARDIAL INFARCTION

1. Insert venous 'access' and admit to monitoring and resuscitation area as quickly as possble
2. Give 2.5-5 mg diamorphine i.v. together with an anti-emetic (e.g. 12.5 mg prochlorperazine)
3. Assess and treat any complications e.g. left ventricular failure or arrhythmias

VENTRICULAR ECTOPICS

Following myocardial infarction, consider treating the V.E. beats when:
1. More than 5 per minute
2. Multifocal origin
3. R on T configuration

Run of 3.

Give lignocaine i.v. bolus 50 mg in 2 min then infusion of 3 mg/min for 1 hour followed by 2 mg/min for several hours gradually reducing to 1 mg/min.

Alternatively disopyramide given as a bolus of 2 mg/kg (not exceeding 150 mg) slowly over 5 min, then infusion of 400 μg/kg/hour (or orally 200 mg 8-hourly).

VENTRICULAR TACHYCARDIA

Cardiovert
If recurrent, start lignocaine or disopyramide.
If arrythmia is resistant, consider i.v. amiodarone.

SINUS BRADYCARDIA

Observe, unless after myocardial infarction and ventricular ectopics escaping, in which case 0.3 mg – 0.6 mg i.v. of atropine may speed up the rate.

HEART BLOCK

1. **First degree heart block**
   Prolonged PR. Observe.

2. **Second degree heart block**
   Mobitz type 1 (Wenckebach) needs no treatment.
   Mobitz type 2 (dropped beats but normal PR) after anterior infarction is more ominous and may need pacing.

3. **Third degree heart block**
   Consider pacing. Pacing is indicated if the infarct is recent, or if Stokes-Adams attacks have occurred. Give isoprenaline while pacing is being organized (2 mg in 500 ml dextrose at 10-30 drops/min to raise ventricular rate above 60 beats/min).

SUPRAVENTRICULAR TACHYCARDIAS

1. Carotid massage
2. Cardiovert if life threatening. Start with 50 joules and increase. If conscious, requires very brief G.A. or i.v. diazepam
3. Verapamil (check not on ß blockers). 5 mg i.v. slowly repeated 5-10 minutes later if no effect
4. Disopyramide or i.v. practolol if no response to verapamil, but allow time for the first agent to clear

ATRIAL FIBRILLATION

Digitalise (digoxin 0.5 mg orally for 3 doses 6-hourly, then 0.25 mg daily according to clinical response and plasma levels). In acute situations, may need to cardiovert (e.g., post-myocardial infarct, where impaired cardiac output threatens myocardium).

ACUTE PULMONARY OEDEMA

1. Sit the patient up in a cardiac bed, with legs dependant, and give oxygen by a high concentration mask
2. Give frusemide 80 mg i.v.
3. Give 2.5-5 mg morphine i.v. slowly to relieve distress
4. Search for and treat any underlying cause e.g. arrhythmia, hypertension, myocardial infarction
5. If no response to above after 45 minutes, repeat diuretic, and give vasodilators, such as glyceryl trinitrate paste or oral prazosin (0.5 mg test then build up t.i.d.s.), long acting nitrates or i.v. or oral hydrallazine. In severe failure consider i.v. nitrates or nitroprusside
6. If patient is exhausted, consider positive pressure ventilation

MASSIVE PULMONARY EMBOLISM

Resuscitate the patient with external cardiac compression, oxygen administration, vasopressor drugs and correction of acidosis as necessary.
   Subsequent therapy depends on the severity of the condition
1. Patients likely to die within an hour or so — bypass embolectomy (if facilities available)
2. Slightly less critically ill patients — streptokinase infusion
3. Milder cases — heparin followed by oral anticoagulants

ACUTE EXACERBATION OF OBSTRUCTIVE AIRWAYS DISEASE

1. Treat any acute infection with antibiotics
2. Relieve hypoxia with controlled oxygen therapy using a Ventimask. Monitor arterial blood gases on each concentration (starting with 24%) and aim to raise PO_2 to greater than 8kPa (60 mmHg) without a rise in PCO_2
3. Vigorous physiotherapy, with assisted coughing
4. Use salbutamol by nebuliser, and if necessary, aminophylline. Consider trial of steroids in case of a reversible element to the obstructive airways disease. Steam inhalations may help to loosen secretions
5. Treat right ventricular failure (cor pulmonale) with diuretics
6. If progressive rise of PCO_2 with increasing narcosis, consider respiratory stimulants or the need for artificial ventilation

N.B. All sedatives must be avoided.

ACUTE ANAPHYLAXIS

The 'shock' is due to:
1. Respiratory obstruction (laryngeal oedema and severe bronchospasm)
2. Circulatory collapse (low plasma volume due to leakage of fluid into interstitial tissues)

In anaphylaxis due to an injection or sting, apply a tourniquet to the injected part as soon as possible.

Hydrocortisone 300 mg i.v. should be given immediately together with 0.5 ml adrenaline (1:1000) *subcutaneously*. The adrenaline should not be repeated, as it may accumulate at the injection site and be absorbed rapidly when the circulation improves. An antihistamine, e.g. promethazine 50 mg i.v. can also be given.

Resuscitation with external cardiac compression, intubation (or tracheostomy) and mechanical ventilation may be required.

Restoration of plasma volume by infusion of fluid may be important, monitored by central venous pressure.

DIABETIC KETOACIDAEMIC COMA

No inflexible rules can be given, since individual patients vary in their requirements. Treatment must be monitored throughout by frequent biochemical and clinical monitoring
1. Identify and treat the precipitating cause, e.g. infection. If no cause is apparent a broad-spectrum antibiotic may be used empirically (after taking blood, sputum and urine for culture)
2. Take blood for glucose, urea and electrolytes, haematocrit and arterial blood pH
3. Infuse N saline — 2 litres in the first 2 hours, then 1 litre every 2 hours. Beware of cardiac failure in old people or those with cardiac disease
4. Give soluble insulin at rate of 5-10 units hourly by constant infusion using automatic pump or deep i.m. injection. Aim to produce a steady fall in blood glucose
5. Potassium 20 mmol/hour should be added to the infusion after the first hour. Replacement should be guided by the blood levels
6. If initial pH is 7.00 or below, give 100 mmol sodium bicarbonate i.v. and repeat plasma sodium and bicarbonate
7. If there is gastric dilatation or vomiting pass a tube and empty the stomach. Bladder catheterization may be required but is not recommended as a routine
8. Check blood glucose, urea and electrolytes 1 hour after the first dose of insulin, and 2-hourly thereafter. If the first post-insulin blood glucose has not fallen significantly the insulin infusion dose is increased
9. When blood glucose reaches 12 mmol/l, replace the saline infusion with 5% dextrose

Continue the insulin infusion and the dextrose until ketosis is corrected, then establish a 6-hourly insulin regime and later adjust to twice daily.

'STATUS EPILEPTICUS'

Establish an adequate airway and give oxygen.

Give 2-15 mg diazepam by slow i.v. injection until convulsions cease. Set up intravenous infusion of diazepam (max. 3 mg/kg/24 h.) Adjust dose to prevent convulsions but beware of respiratory depression. If venepuncture is impossible give 10 mg i.m. A suitable alternative is paraldehyde (5 ml into each of 2 i.m. sites, using a glass syringe). Failure to control seizures is an indication for curarisation and ventilation. Seek and treat any cause for fits particularly infection (eg. meningitis). Take blood for calcium, magnesium and glucose estimation and give 50 ml of 50% glucose i.v. to exclude hypoglycaemia.

Start prophylaxis as soon as possible. Give phenytoin 300 mg orally 8-hourly for 1 day then 300 mg daily. Adjust dose according to response and plasma drug levels.

SEVERE ASTHMA

Administer oxygen with a Ventimask (35%).

Administer salbutamol 2.5-5 mg by inhalation from a nebulizer 4-6 hourly. If severe, administer 250 μg by slow i.v. infusion. Give hydrocortisone 300 mg i.v. followed by 200 mg 4-hourly. Oral prednisolone (40 mg/day) should start on the same day. Consider aminophylline 250-500 mg by slow i.v. injection after checking the patient has not taken oral theophylline. Always give with oxygen, and monitor for arrythmias. If severe, maintain aminophylline infusion at a rate of 9 mg/kg/24 hours. Never sedate. Check the arterial blood gases, and assess the response to treatment by serial analysis.

Exclude pneumothorax by X-ray. Start broad-spectrum antibiotics after blood and sputum cultures (e.g. tetracycline, ampicillin or Septrin). Correct dehydration (if necessary use i.v. fluids). Watch for danger signs of exhaustion, inability to speak or cough, impaired consciousness, rising pulse rate or increasing pulse paradox, rising temperature and worsening blood gases (rising PCO_2 and falling PO_2). In very severe cases, consider mechanical ventilation.

ACUTE GASTROINTESTINAL HAEMORRHAGE

1. Treat shock with i.v. plasma or Haemacell while awaiting blood
2. Elevate foot of bed and give oxygen. If distressed give small dose of sedative
3. Monitor the central venous pressure to prevent over-transfusion and to detect rebleeding
4. Determine the cause of haemorrhage (endoscopy or Ba meal according to facilities)
5. Start cimetidine and antacids
6. If bleeding from oesophageal varices, and it fails to stop, consider i.v. vasopressin (20 units in 100 ml 5% dextrose over 15 min) or Sengstaken tube
7. If rebleeds or fails to stop, continue to resuscitate and consider emergency surgery

MANAGEMENT OF ACUTE POISONING

General principles

1. *Prevent further absorption:*
   Stomach washout is advisable except in the following
   circumstances:
   (i) Corrosive and oil-based poisons
   (ii) Drowsy or comatose patients (unless a cuffed endotracheal
       tube is used)
   (iii) Delay of 4 hr or more after ingestion (except after salicylates
        or tricyclics, or if taken with alcohol, in which stomach
        emptying is delayed)
2. *Intensive supportive treatment:*
   (i) Nurse prone and clear the airways
   (ii) Use artificial ventilation if minute volume is less than 4 litres
   (iii) Maintain hydration
   (iv)   Treat hyper- or hypothermia
   (v) Monitor heart rate, blood pressure, peripheral perfusion and
       urine output
   (vi) Treat convulsions and arrhythmias
3. *Antidotes and elimination of poison:*
   (i) Forced alkaline diuresis for weak acids, e.g. salicylates
   (ii) Dialysis is rarely useful, since most drugs do not dialyse
       freely
   (iii) Specific antidotes, e.g. naloxone for morphine
   (iv) For unfamiliar drugs or toxins contact your Poisons Information
       Centre:
   Tel. London (01)-407 7600
        Edinburgh (031)-229 2477
        Cardiff (0222)-49 2233
        Belfast (0232)-24 0503

Barbiturates
Intensive supportive treatment
Forced diuresis should be considered for phenobarbitone

Salicylates
Absorption is slow, therefore stomach washout is advisable.
   Expect complicated metabolic disturbances, e.g. respiratory
alkalosis, metabolic acidosis and hypoprothrombinaemia.
   Forced alkaline diuresis is very effective, but dangerous in elderly
and in cardiac or renal failure, or if not properly monitored.
   Blood salicylate level is a good guide to severity of poisoning.
   Use forced alkaline diuresis if level greater than 450 mg/l.

Ethanol
Prevention of aspiration of vomitus is important.
  In severe cases gastric lavage is needed, with supportive therapy as required (artificial ventilation, etc.).
  In very severe poisoning, peritoneal dialysis or haemodialysis is indicated.

Iron salts
High mortality in children if untreated. Symptoms are GI irritation, dehydration and delayed damage to liver and c.n.s.
  Empty the stomach immediately by inducing vomiting and follow with gastric lavage using desferrioxamine solution (2 g in 1 litre). Leave 10 g desferrioxamine in 50 ml water in the stomach and give 2 g of desferrioxamine i.m.

Carbon monoxide
Remove the patient from the poisonous atmosphere, clear the airway and give artificial respiration with 100% oxygen with the patient prone.
  After spontaneous breathing starts there may be relapse into coma due to cerebral oedema, which may require i.v. infusion of 500 ml of 20% mannitol.
  Anoxic heart or brain damage may occur.

Narcotics (morphine, etc.)
Hypoventilation should be treated with naloxone 0.4 mg i.v. which acts within 2 min and may be repeated at 3 min intervals.

Phenothiazines
Little disturbance of consciousness and respiratory depression, but drugs for convulsions and cardiac arrhythmias may be needed.

Tricyclic antidepressives
These cause dry mouth, dilated pupils, disturbed consciousness, cardiac arrhythmias and in severe cases respiratory failure and hypotension. E.c.g. monitoring is advisable. Physostigmine 1-3 mg i.v. over 2 min will reverse c.n.s. effects and will counteract some cardiac effects.

Amphetamines
These cause hyperactivity and psychosis, followed by exhaustion, convulsions, hyperthermia and coma.
  Barbiturates counteract the early stages and later anticonvulsants, cooling and artificial ventilation may be required.

Bleaching agents
These are highly irritant. Gastric lavage is advisable, and milk and aluminium hydroxide gel should be given.

Dry cleaning fluids (C Cl₄, etc)

If inhaled, artificial ventilation may be needed.
If swallowed, gastric lavage is required.
Acute hepatic and renal failure may follow.

Petroleum products and paraffin (kerosene)

Gastric lavage is contraindicted because aspiration of a small
amount causes pneumonitis. Absorption from the stomach is
slowed by giving 250 ml of liquid paraffin.

Cyanide

Speed is essential. Inject two 20 ml ampoules of 1.5% dicobalt
tetracemate (Kelocyanor) intravenously, followed by 20 ml of 50%
glucose.

Gastric lavage and artificial ventilation with oxygen are also
recommended.

Mouth-to-mouth resuscitation can be dangerous for the doctor or
nurse because of the risk of contamination with cyanide.

Paracetamol

A toxic metabolite causes hepatic damage within 4 days. Oral
methionine or i.v. cysteamine may prevent this damage if given
within 10 hours of ingestion.

Measure plasma levels at or after 4 hours from ingestion:

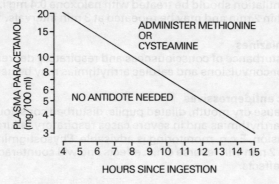

Index

151